POSITIVE COOKING

LISA McMILLAN, RD
JILL JARVIE, RD, CNSD
JANET BRAUER

Avery Publishing Group
Garden City Park, New York

Text Illustrator: John Wincek
Cover Design: Rudy Shur and William Gonzalez
Cover Photo: Bill Dobos, H. Armstrong Roberts
Typesetter: Bonnie Freid
In-House Editor: Lisa James
Printer: Paragon Press, Honesdale, PA

Library of Congress Cataloging-in-Publication Data

McMillan, Lisa.
    Positive cooking : cooking for people living with HIV / by Lisa
McMillan, Jill Jarvie, Janet Brauer.
       p. cm.
    Includes bibliographical references and index.
    ISBN 0-89529-734-5
    1. AIDS (Disease)—Diet therapy—Recipes. 2. AIDS (Disease)-
-Nutritional aspects. I. Jarvie, Jill. II. Brauer, Janet.
III. Title.
RC607.A26M394 1997
616.97'920654—DC20   96-33390
                                CIP

Printed in the United States of America

10 9 8 7 6 5 4 3 2 1

Contents

This book is lovingly dedicated to our family and friends,
and all those touched by HIV disease.

Acknowledgments

We were very fortunate to receive the generous assistance of a great many people while completing this book. In particular, we owe our sincere gratitude and appreciation to Rudy Shur and Avery Publishing for giving us the opportunity to publish this book, and for patiently walking us through the process. We also owe gratitude to our clients and friends at Project Open Hand in San Francisco, who have taught us so much about living with HIV disease; to Karen Frank and Tom Clynes, who were there at the beginning with counsel and advice; and to Geoff Frampton and Pat Rooney, who donated their hardware and are sources of ongoing support. We wish to thank Lee Weinstein, Vaughn Welty, and Jamie Horwitz, who provided useful input and resources, and Bert Bloom, Colleen Martin, and Michele McMahon, who have provided valuable feedback on the content of the book. Thank you to Tommy Baranauskas and Jeff Davis, who provided the technical support we needed to troubleshoot along the way. We gratefully acknowledge Marc K. Hellerstein, M.D., Ph.D., who has not only contributed to this book, but who continues to do important work in the AIDS community.

We offer special thanks to our tasters—Mathew Atlee, Irene Romano, Carol Ohnstad, and Danny Vuic—for making sure we got it right, and to our friends and families for their constant support, helpful feedback, and wonderful recipes.

We also wish to thank Stephen (Chief) Schneider for his ongoing counsel and endless encouragement. We could not have done it without you.

ACKNOWLEDGMENTS

Foreword

Imagine the following: there's an epidemic condition that alters the nutritional state of almost everyone affected. The condition is associated with a wide range of symptoms and—most important—with shortened survival. But there are also the means to address these symptoms, maintain health, and improve quality of life, and there are experts on this subject who want to share their enormous experience. Wouldn't you want to hear what they have to say?

Positive Cooking, a cookbook and nutrition guide, provides that opportunity for people with HIV disease. I've been involved in research on the causes and treatment of weight loss associated with HIV infection for quite a while, and I know of no one more qualified to write such a book than these authors. Dietitians Lisa McMillan and Jill Jarvie have accumulated unequaled hands-on experience in counseling and feeding people with HIV and AIDS. McMillan works for Project Open Hand, the San Francisco-based organization that provides meals for the greatest number of HIV-infected people of any nutrition program in the world—approximately 600,000 meals for about 4,500 people a year. Jarvie, who used to work at Open Hand, works for the San Francisco Department of Public Health. And Janet Brauer has broad experience in writing about nutrition and HIV from her work with Project Open Hand, including work on publications such as *Positive Nutrition*, a nationally distributed newsletter on HIV and nutrition. The combination of these talents results in expert dietary advice presented in a clear and concise manner.

This book contains a wealth of detailed information to help anyone with HIV infection. There are pearls of advice that address nutritional problems specific to people with HIV infection, such as the peculiarities of taste that sometimes arise, or tips on food safety, or how to deal with mouth discomfort and chronic diarrhea without compromising food intake. Moreover, as important as the many specific tips and pieces of advice is the philosophy that informs the book. The authors recognize the importance of preventing weight loss and its consequent effect on health, rather than waiting for weight loss to occur before taking action.

Recent research in the history of AIDS-associated body wasting strongly supports this preventative perspective. If one looks closely at the pattern of weight loss in AIDS, it becomes apparent that most people lose weight in spurts. An episode of sickness is accompanied by loss of appetite and a bout of rapid weight loss; during recovery the weight is only partially regained. Worse, the weight lost may disproportionately represent lean tissue, while the weight regained later may tilt toward fat. These research findings have potentially important implications for anyone hoping to prevent weight loss. Might it be possible to short-circuit lean tissue wasting by maintaining good food intake during bouts of illness? This is a difficult challenge for the patient, but many of the tips in this book may help to at least minimize the extent of each bout of weight loss and to maximize gains during each recovery phase.

Reading this book reminds me how much is known about HIV and nutrition, but also how much still remains mysterious. Why do people lose their appetite when they get sick? Why does the body's metabolism change and seem to favor body fat over lean tissue? Who should receive additional intensive therapies such as growth hormone, appetite stimulants, and hormone replacement? These and other questions do not yet have definite scientific answers.

In the meantime, people have to live and make decisions.

Positive Cooking contains many precepts, carefully laid out, to help individuals with HIV help themselves. The authors recommend the formation of a health care team for each individual that includes people such as health care providers, dietitians, and caregivers. This team-building can have many benefits. It can help promote early recognition and treatment of emerging infections, which may prevent severe or prolonged spells of weight loss. And reporting symptoms that suggest hormone deficiencies to one's physician may allow appropriate replacement therapy.

The book also covers other topics. Careful selection of foods or supplements that do not worsen gastrointestinal symptoms may allow weight main-

tenance even in the presence of chronic diarrhea. Exercise may help preserve lean tissue. Stress reduction can improve both eating habits and overall health.

In my various roles, including work in an undergraduate teaching and graduate research department (at the University of California at Berkeley) and a county hospital (San Francisco General Hospital, which is part of the University of California, San Francisco), I've had the privilege of working with a wide spectrum of students and colleagues. They range from undergraduates to graduate students, medical students, housestaff, fellows, and faculty of basic sciences and medicine. As strong a respect as I have for any of these groups, I hold as much or more for people on the front lines of patient care and prevention. I consider the authors of this book to be in the latter category. It is my honor to write a foreword to their book. It is the reader's good fortune to have access to their insight and experience.

Marc K. Hellerstein, M.D., Ph.D.

Associate Professor,
Department of Nutritional Sciences,
University of California at Berkeley

Associate Professor, Division of
Endocrinology and Metabolism,
Department of Medicine,
San Francisco General Hospital,
University of California,
San Francisco

Preface

For most of us, throughout our lives, food is the constant that provides us with comfort, draws us together in celebration and support, and nourishes our spirit, all while satisfying our hunger. In times of illness, as the body's nutritional needs are significantly altered, food takes on an even more important role in maintaining health and emotional well-being.

Research has uncovered a great deal of information about the critical link between nutrition and the well-being of people living with HIV disease. As part of our work—providing nutrition counseling to individuals and writing a nationally distributed newsletter—we spent countless hours examining this information. We found that many people with HIV—and their caregivers, families, and friends—knew very little about the specific nutritional needs of a person living with HIV and, more importantly, knew little about how to meet those needs. We were asked a lot of questions.

I'm a person living with HIV disease. I know I need to gain weight, but recently I just don't seem to have the energy to cook a big dinner. What can I eat that will put on weight, but is easy to prepare?

My brother has AIDS and I live with him now to help out. It's easier for me to make one dinner for the two of us. Is it all right to still cook our favorite meal of turkey, mashed potatoes, and gravy?

My medications make me so nauseated I don't feel like eating. How can I decrease my nausea and get my appetite back?

We wrote *Positive Cooking* because many of our clients and friends were looking for basic, easy-to-follow nutrition advice to help restore or maintain their quality of life. We found that much of the information available was either geared toward the scientific community or was not specific to HIV disease and, therefore, was consistently incorrect and dangerously misleading for people with HIV. For instance, most mainstream-media nutrition stories focus on persuading people to *lose* weight. With malnutrition occurring in at least 87 percent of the population with HIV, there is an overwhelming need for information and education on how to help *maintain* or *increase* weight.

We also wanted to stress the importance of nutrition awareness for individuals at every stage of the disease—whether they have symptoms or not. Early nutrition planning in order to prevent malnutrition and body wasting is critical to everyone who lives with HIV disease.

In addition, clients were asking for specific recipes to address specific symptoms, and we found ourselves constantly scrambling to come up with suitable choices. There was no resource like *Positive Cooking* available.

Our goal was to provide a relatively easy-to-follow, practical guide to nutrition and HIV, along with some truly tempting and nourishing recipes specifically chosen for people living with this disease. We hope you will use this book as a practical tool to help meet your nutrition needs, and that you will continue to educate yourself as more information becomes available (see the Resource List).

We also encourage you to get involved with an AIDS care provider in your community. Go deliver meals, chop vegetables, answer phones, contribute whatever you can financially, and cook these recipes for friends and family. We guarantee that the rewards will be tremendous!

Introduction

It's during times of illness or stress that the body requires the most nourishment to thrive. We know there is a critical link between nutrition and HIV disease. We also know that the enjoyment one derives from food should not diminish simply because one is ill. Meals designed to meet your nutritional needs can be truly satisfying and thoroughly enjoyable. The recipes in this book will not remind you of hospital fare. Rather, they are some of our tastiest triumphs in the kitchen.

In addition to serving as an everyday cookbook, this book provides guidelines to help a person living with HIV meet specific nutrition requirements. Those who care for people living with HIV will also find this book, which includes information on meal planning and preparation, to be an important resource. And there are practical tips on how to help ease the most commonly experienced symptoms associated with HIV disease.

The first section in Part One, Treating HIV Disease with Chicken Soup, begins with a discussion on the importance of nutrition in treatment and then gives a brief overview of basic nutrition. The second section, Health Management and HIV, outlines specific nutrition recommendations for people with HIV. These recommendations are illustrated by a food guide, specially developed for people with HIV, which shows how much of what food types should be eaten each day. You will also find a quick reference table that gives vitamin and mineral supplement recommendations. In addition, you will find information on food and water safety, which is extremely important in reducing the risk of contracting food- or water-borne illness. There is also information for caregivers.

Each individual's nutritional needs will vary during the course of his or her HIV infection. Therefore, we feel it is of great importance to provide nutrition tips that address the most commonly experienced symptoms. In the section Using Diet to Help Alleviate HIV Symptoms, you will find practical information on adapting to problems related to the mouth and throat, and on improving appetite, controlling constipation, decreasing diarrhea, fighting fatigue, alleviating nausea and vomiting, and gaining or maintaining weight in the form of lean body mass. At the end of the information provided for each symptom, you will find a seven-day meal plan for that specific symptom.

Part Two consists of recipes designed to address the specific nutritional needs of someone living with HIV. We have focused on providing recipes that are not only enticing and soothing, but are also easy to make and contain ingredients most people would keep on hand. We chose many of these recipes because they were our childhood favorites, or were the traditional comfort foods of relatives and friends. Each recipe contains a calorie count, and the amounts of carbohydrates, protein, and fat. Each recipe also lists the symptoms that recipe is designed to alleviate.

Because many individuals experience more than one symptom at the same time during the course of an HIV infection, you will find easy-to-follow recipe-by-symptoms charts at the beginning of each recipe section. The charts allow for cross-referencing between symptoms and recipes designed to help address those symptoms. For instance, if both fatigue and loss of appetite are problems, the chart in the Main Fare section will tell you which entrée recipes can help alleviate both symptoms.

How have these recipes been designed to help someone with HIV adapt to various symptoms? The recipes designed for chewing and swallowing difficulties, dry mouth, and mouth and throat sores include foods that are soothing, soft, moist, and easy to chew. The recipes for alterations in taste contain flavors that spark the taste buds, including citrus or tangy flavors. The recipes intended to alleviate loss of appetite provide smaller servings that are high in calories and protein. The recipes designed to control constipation are high in fiber, containing at least 10 grams of dietary fiber per entrée and 5 grams of dietary fiber per snack or side dish. The recipes intended to help relieve diarrhea are low in fat and insoluble fiber, and are lactose- and caffeine-free. For fatigue, we have chosen recipes that are high in complex carbohydrates and protein for energy, and

either are easy to prepare or can be prepared in advance and frozen for later use. The recipes designed to help ease nausea and vomiting are low in fat, with mild seasonings. The recipes chosen to help a person gain weight provide larger servings, and emphasize calories from carbohydrates and protein.

As you would with any cookbook, we encourage you to experiment with ingredients and spices to match your tolerances and meet your tastes. It's also important to remember you don't always need to eat a breakfast food for breakfast or an entrée for your main meal. As long as you're meeting your daily nutritional requirements, you may find you prefer to eat breakfast for dinner or vice versa. Consult a registered dietitian with questions about meeting your specific nutritional requirements.

Sprinkled throughout the recipe sections are directions for cooking various basic foods. There are also some basic cooking terms in the introduction to Part Two, and a Resource List at the back of the book to help you find out all you can about nutrition and HIV disease.

We've spent the last several years researching the information provided in this book, and have seen the encouraging results nutrition management has brought to the lives of our clients and friends. Nutrition management is a cost-effective treatment you can begin immediately with guidance from a registered dietitian. As you continue to use the information and recipes provided in this book, we hope you will begin to see the difference in your quality of life.

Enjoy!

Part One

Basic Information

Each person with HIV has particular nutritional needs and, therefore, needs an individualized approach to treatment. In this part, we provide background material on the connection between HIV and nutrition to help you understand the individual nutrition goals that you should be working toward. There is some information on basic nutrition and the immune system, along with specific daily nutrition requirements for people living with HIV. There are recommendations for building a team of health professionals and for actively participating in your health care, especially in the area of nutrition. The important topic of food and water safety is covered. And there are tips and meal plans you can use to help alleviate common symptoms, such as fatigue and appetite loss, that often accompany an HIV infection. This information is intended to help you understand the principles upon which the recipes in Part Two are based.

Treating HIV Disease With Chicken Soup

Many of us grew up hearing the sage advice, "Eat this, you'll feel better." For a person living with human immunodeficiency virus (HIV), or with any chronic illness, this statement is particularly true. After years of research into effective, reliable remedies for HIV disease, medical experts are finally acknowledging an invaluable treatment: chicken soup.

A nutritionally sound diet can play an important role in helping a person living with HIV disease improve or maintain health. Such a diet should include comforting, familiar foods such as chicken soup, corn bread, and meat loaf, as well as many other recipes you will find in this book.

Someone living with HIV disease must develop a healthy, nutritious diet as soon as the infection is discovered, and should maintain a sound nutrition regimen throughout the course of the disease. Not only can good nutrition help combat the many common symptoms associated with HIV disease, but it can also help maintain the health of an HIV-positive person who has no symptoms. Some research suggests that a person's nutritional state may be even more important to overall health than his or her level of immune function, and that survival and longevity may be determined more by a person's nutritional state than by the presence of any particular opportunistic infection.

Proper nutrition can help strengthen the immune system. It can also help:

- Prevent malnutrition and body wasting
- Enhance the body's ability to fight opportunistic infections
- Maintain body weight and strength
- Slow or prevent the breakdown of body tissues
- Improve or support emotional well-being
- Boost energy
- Enhance the body's ability to cope with medical treatments
- Improve the effectiveness of drug treatments

The goal of good nutrition is to maintain a well-balanced diet. "Balanced" means a diet that includes a variety of foods. Such variety provides the full range of vitamins, minerals, carbohydrates, proteins, fats, and other nutrients necessary both to help maintain health and weight, and to prevent vitamin and mineral deficiencies.

Working with your health care professional to design a well-balanced diet tailored to meet your specific needs is an immediate, affordable, and active way to take control of your overall health and treatment. It's never too soon to start learning all you can about nutrition and HIV.

You can get started by reading the following material on the immune system, malnutrition, body wasting, and good-nutrition basics. You will find specific recommendations and a food guide, both designed to meet the needs of people with HIV, in the section Health Management and HIV. You can also get more information from the organizations listed in the Resource Guide.

THE IMMUNE SYSTEM AND HIV

There is a strong relationship between nutrition and the immune system. The immune system's function is to defend the body against invaders such as bacteria, viruses, fungi, and parasites. Good nutrition plays an important role in building and maintaining a strong immune system by providing the body with the nutrients it needs to help fight off disease and infection, and to combat symptoms. In a healthy person, the immune system operates through a system of checks and balances, passing information back and forth in an elaborate communications network that produces an immune response. Immune response is the body's ability to recognize and eliminate foreign materials—to distinguish between self and non-self.

An immune deficiency disorder, such as HIV, occurs when one or more of the immune system's components are lacking. In the case of HIV, the virus destroys the small white blood cells, called T4 cells, that orchestrate and participate in the immune response. Therefore, the immune system is not able to correctly identify foreign invaders, and the immune response is misguided.

As a result, HIV disease is characterized by a variety of unusual infections. These infections are known as "opportunistic" infections because they are produced by commonplace organisms that would not normally affect a healthy individual, but take advantage of the "opportunity" presented by a damaged immune system.

MALNUTRITION AND THE PROGRESSION OF HIV

Malnutrition occurs when the body can't get enough of the nutrients it needs to maintain good health. It is a common and important complication of HIV disease—at least 67 percent of people with HIV and 87 percent of people with AIDS are malnourished. Malnutrition and the complications that it causes can put significant stress on the immune system by contributing to the development of opportunistic infections, reducing the effectiveness of medications, hindering the absorption of nutrients from the intestines, and reducing the quality of life. This stress, in turn, can hasten the progression of HIV disease and shorten survival time.

Inadequate calories, protein, vitamins, and minerals may all lead to malnutrition. People with HIV may develop malnutrition for a number of reasons:

- They may eat less
- Their intestines may not be able to properly absorb nutrients from food
- Their bodies may use up energy supplies more quickly than normal—or may not use energy as efficiently—because of the energy needed to fight the disease, especially in the presence of opportunistic infections

Opportunistic infections, medication side effects, stress, depression, and cancers associated with HIV can all produce symptoms and result in special dietary needs that may contribute to malnutrition. The symptoms that occur most often are:

- Mouth and throat complications, including sores, alterations in taste, dry mouth, and difficulty in chewing and swallowing
- Loss of appetite
- Constipation
- Diarrhea
- Fatigue
- Nausea and vomiting
- Weight loss or body wasting

For specific tips and recipes designed to help address each of these symptoms, refer to the section Using Diet to Help Alleviate HIV Symptoms, and to the recipe-by-symptoms charts at the beginning of each Part Two section.

BODY WASTING AND THE NEED TO BUILD MUSCLE

A big problem that confronts people with HIV is body wasting. The Centers for Disease Control (CDC) defines body wasting as loss of more than 10 percent of usual body weight accompanied by either chronic diarrhea—diarrhea that lasts more than thirty days—or chronic weakness and fever, when there is no illness or condition other than HIV that would produce such symptoms. Body wasting is accompanied by an accelerated loss of lean body mass, which mostly consists of muscle. The HIV wasting syndrome was named by the CDC in 1987 as an AIDS-defining illness.

HIV wasting syndrome differs from starvation in that in wasting it is lean body mass—protein—that is broken down and used for energy instead of fat. Research has shown that in many cases people with HIV disease may be dying of malnutrition and body wasting, rather than of the direct effects of infection or malignancy.

Malnutrition and opportunistic infections can be major causes of body wasting. While the first step should be to treat any opportunistic infections present, the next and equally important step is to develop a balanced diet that will supply the body with the many nutrients it needs to build lean body mass and prevent breakdown of body tissue. The loss of lean body mass, which consists mostly of muscle, harms health more than the weight loss itself.

Decreases in body weight, in body fat, and in lean body mass have been seen in patients in the early stages of HIV infection. This indicates that people with HIV should focus on nutrition before malnutrition and weight loss become severe. It is much easier to prevent weight loss and malnutrition than it is to regain lost ground.

Because it may be difficult to recognize or identify early weight loss, it is important for you to monitor your weight (see the weight chart on page 25). If there is continued weight loss, your health care professional, such as a registered dietitian, should be notified. The causes of weight loss may vary, so different approaches to treatment may be recommended. Weight loss from diarrhea, for instance, may require a different strategy than weight loss from loss of appetite. Anabolic agents such as growth hormones and testosterone can be used to treat body wasting in some people. A health care professional can provide information about these medications, and about effective exercise programs designed to increase lean body mass.

THE BASICS OF GOOD NUTRITION

"You are what you eat." Sound familiar? The foods you eat are made up of many different kinds of materials. Water is the most plentiful, followed by such solids as carbohydrate, protein, and fat. The human body is also made up of these very same materials.

Nutrition is the taking in of nourishment—food—necessary for life. Generally, the best way to get the nutrients your body needs is to eat a wide variety of foods. Whole grains, lean proteins, fruits, and vegetables should be emphasized, with less emphasis on sugar, fats, oils, and processed foods.

Food is the fuel that gives your body energy and the ability to function and grow. The body uses nutrients obtained from food to promote growth, maintenance, and repair. Nutrients can be divided into two categories: energy nutrients and nonenergy nutrients.

The Energy Nutrients

The body is a collection of molecules that move. The energy nutrients—carbohydrates, fats, and proteins—give the body the ability to move. Calories measure the amount of energy foods release when burned. When we talk about the calorie content of a food, we are referring to the amount of carbohydrates, fat, and protein it contains.

Carbohydrates

Carbohydrates are the main source of energy for the body, supplying this energy in the form of glucose, which is also referred to as blood sugar. There are two classes of carbohydrates, the complex carbohydrates and the simple carbohydrates.

Complex carbohydrates are primarily starches. The main sources of complex carbohydrates include grain-based foods such as bread, cereals, rice, and pasta, and vegetables such as potatoes and corn. Foods high in starch tend to be low in fat, and provide a better balance of nutrients than foods high in sugar.

Simple carbohydrates are the sugars. There are many forms of sugar, including white table sugar, honey, corn syrup, molasses, and fruit juice. While simple carbohydrates do provide calories, they do not provide the body with the other nutrients it needs.

Proteins

All proteins are various combinations of twenty-two amino acids. Although our bodies make some amino acids, there are others that can only be obtained from food. These are known as essential amino acids, in that it is essential that they be included in the diet.

Complete proteins contain all the essential amino acids. Animal proteins, such as those found in meat, poultry, fish, eggs, and dairy products, are naturally complete proteins.

Plant-based proteins are called incomplete proteins because they lack, or have limited amounts of, one or more of the essential amino acids. Peas and beans, tofu, nuts, seeds, and grain products such as rice, noodles, cereals, and bread are examples of incomplete proteins. You can, however, combine incomplete proteins to make complete proteins. Examples of such protein pairings include serving beans with rice or tortillas, vegetarian chili with corn bread, and hummus with whole wheat pita bread. Because the body stores protein for later use, you do not have to eat a complete protein at every meal as long as you eat proteins that complement one another throughout the day.

Fats

When we talk about fats, we are referring to both fats and oils. We can divide fats into:

- Saturated fats, which come mainly from animal sources such as dairy products and meat, but also include coconut and palm oils
- Polyunsaturated fats, which include safflower, corn, and sesame oils
- Monounsaturated fats, which include canola, olive, peanut, and avocado oils

Fats are necessary to good health. Fat helps maintain the health of skin and hair, protects body organs, helps transport fat-soluble vitamins, and provides a reserve fuel supply in healthy individuals. Most persons can get the fat their body needs directly from a well-balanced diet without adding fats such as butter, margarine, or mayonnaise to their meals.

It's important to keep in mind that both the type and amount of fat consumed can affect your health. For instance, too much saturated fat in your diet may increase the risk of heart disease and tends to raise overall cholesterol levels. It's generally recommended that more of the fat in one's diet should come from monounsaturated and polyunsaturated fats, because these types of fat pose fewer health risks.

The Nonenergy Nutrients

Water, vitamins, and minerals are nutrients that do not directly provide energy. However, they are necessary to keep various bodily functions, such as energy production and digestion, running smoothly. They also allow the body to produce healthy bones, teeth, skin, and blood.

Water

Water is the most essential nutrient—it makes up 55 to 60 percent of the body's weight. Water performs some extremely important functions in the body, such as carrying nutrients, oxygen, and waste products; acting as part of the chemical structure of cells, tissues, and organs; providing a protective environment for cells, organs, and joints; and regulating body temperature.

Vitamins and Minerals

Vitamins are essential nutrients that are "vital" to life. They help maintain various bodily functions, such as eyesight, blood formation and clotting, and bone and tooth formation. Vitamins also play a vital role in immune response and energy production.

There are two groups of vitamins, those that dissolve in water and those that dissolve in fat. Water-soluble vitamins are absorbed into the blood. The B-complex vitamins and vitamin C are examples of water-soluble vitamins. The body uses as much of the water-soluble vitamins as it needs that day, then rids itself of the excess by passing it out in the urine. Since the body can't store these vitamins, they must be consumed in small amounts every day.

Fat-soluble vitamins cannot be absorbed directly into the bloodstream, but instead must be carried by fats. Vitamins A, D, E, and K are examples of fat-soluble vitamins. The body can store these vitamins because they are not passed out of the body in the urine. This means an excess of these vitamins may be consumed one day, and the body will store that amount for use at a later date. However, when taken in excess, this storage of vitamins increases the risk of harmful side effects.

Minerals are natural elements that are also essential for proper bodily functioning, including the immune response. The amount of each mineral needed in the diet varies, generally in proportion to the amount of that mineral found in the body. Minerals used by the body include zinc, selenium, calcium, iron, and copper.

The best way to obtain most of the vitamins and minerals your body requires is through food. However, supplements may prove helpful for a person living with HIV disease. For further discussion of this topic, see page 17.

Antioxidants

Antioxidants, which include some vitamins and minerals, neutralize harmful molecules in the body known as free radicals. The body continuously creates free radicals through normal cell functioning and through exposure to sunlight, tobacco smoke, pollution, ozone, and X rays. Free radicals put stress on the immune system because they can damage various cell parts, or even kill cells outright. Examples of antioxidants include beta-carotene, vitamin E, vitamin C, selenium, and zinc.

THE KEYS TO HEALTH

By learning more about basic nutrition and about the best ways to nourish the body, you are already well on your way to meeting what should be one of your first nutrition goals—discovering all you can about the importance of nutrition in the treatment of HIV disease. Remember the keys to a healthier life with HIV:

- Practicing good nutrition as soon as you learn that you are HIV-positive
- Continuing to monitor your nutritional needs as time goes on, including careful weight checks (see page 24)

To stay healthy, a person with HIV must eat healthy, nutritious foods, foods that will allow him or her to maintain or increase lean body mass. Good nutrition can also help a person manage both the symptoms that often occur with HIV disease and the effects of medical treatment.

Health Management and HIV

Because each person with HIV has different complications and symptoms, treatment plans will vary from person to person. Consequently, it is essential that you take an active role in managing your health. This should be done in partnership with health care professionals as soon as the diagnosis is made, and continued throughout the course of the disease. Remember that it's much easier to maintain weight and strength than it is to recover lost ground.

What does health management mean? Besides teaming up with health care professionals, it means planning for good nutrition, developing an exercise program, reducing and controlling stress, and learning about food and water safety.

While it is important to learn about nutrition, exercise, and stress management, it may not be necessary for you to make broad lifestyle and eating-habit changes all at once. It may be a better idea to set short-term, realistic goals that will help you make more permanent changes over time. (Also, see the inset "Changing Unhealthy Habits" on page 28.)

THE TEAM APPROACH TO GOOD HEALTH

It is important for you to build a team of health care professionals with whom you feel comfortable and who can work with you to help plan your treatment. This team may include a primary care provider, a registered dietitian, a caregiver to help you at home (caregivers should see "Tips for Caregivers" on page 12), a social worker or case manager, a mental health care provider, a fitness trainer, and a dentist. It may also include other care providers, such as an acupuncturist, an herbalist, a chiropractor, or a body worker.

Find individuals who specialize in HIV care. You can find lists of such individuals through patient advocacy groups, your local hospital, your city's health department, or your local AIDS organizations (see the Resource List).

Determine if a prospective health care professional, such as a dietitian, fits well with your personality. If the person works in a clinic setting, get to know the staff members and their habits. Will someone be available to answer any questions you may have during the visit, or between visits on the phone? Will that person be able to explain medical terms and treatments in language you understand?

Developing good communication channels with your health care team is very important, but it may take some time. Prepare for your appointments. Talk to your health care professional about any questions

Tips for Caregivers

It is likely that a person living with HIV disease will need, or find it helpful, to seek some type of assistance from a caregiver at various times throughout his or her illness. Caregiving can range from the informal help provided by family and friends to the formal support of trained medical workers, home care aides, or social workers. The role and duties of a caregiver may vary depending on that person's availability and skills, as well as upon the needs of the person for whom they are caring and the availability of additional resources. As someone who may spend more time with the HIV-positive person than that person's primary health care provider, the caregiver is an important and often vital member of the health care team.

If you are caring for someone with HIV, you can play an important role in health management and nutrition planning. Here are some ways to help:

• Be an active listener. Don't assume that you know exactly what care is needed or wanted. You and the person you're caring for should work together to assess his or her needs and to determine what services you can provide.

• Know your limits. Be fair to yourself and to the person for whom you're caring by setting realistic goals for both of you. Reassess your role and duties every six months, or as needed.

• Be supportive. Respect the decisions and privacy of the person for whom you are providing care. Ultimately, it's not your job to determine what's best for that person and what nutrition program he or she should follow. The individual with HIV is the person responsible for making final decisions on his or her health. Consult a social worker, case manager, or health care professional to help resolve a difficult or health-threatening situation.

• Help with weekly meal planning and grocery shopping. See the shopping and storage safety tips that begin on page 29.

• Help with food preparation. Prewash fruits and vegetables. Chop, slice, dice, or otherwise prepare ingredients ahead of time, and store in airtight, refrigerated containers. Prepare individual servings of foods ahead of time and store them for future use, following the storage and preparation safety tips that start on page 29.

• Help with cleanup. You can also organize supplies, such as by cleaning old food out of the refrigerator and by organizing the pantry.

• Provide company at meals. Good company helps maintain a stress-free environment, and may stimulate appetite.

• Provide a change in surroundings. Offer to take the person you're caring for to a suitable restaurant, or help plan a picnic at a park. A change in surroundings may also help stimulate appetite, and may help improve emotional well-being.

• Help the person you're caring for chart weight and keep a food diary (see page 17).

• Help find needed resources. You will want to work with the person for whom you are providing care, as well as with other members of the health care team. For example, if the team decides that the use of a fitness trainer would be a good idea, call community AIDS or HIV organizations to obtain referrals. Often, helping to make phone calls reduces stress and speeds the process along.

• Assist in coordinating the health care team. Help the person you're caring for keep a day planner to schedule necessary appointments. Record the names and phone numbers of other team members for easy access, and clearly identify the role of each person on the list, such as primary health care provider, registered dietitian, and social worker or case manager. This will prove especially helpful in the event of an emergency.

• Take care of yourself! As a caregiver, it is often easy to forget to attend to your own needs. If you are not at your best, you are not providing the best care possible. Recognize when you need to take a break and reenergize. There are books, tapes, and workshops available to help caregivers cope with the often unavoidable stress that accompanies HIV disease—call your local AIDS or HIV organization for referrals.

you may have regarding your health status and treatment. It may be helpful to bring in a written list of questions and concerns. Don't leave until your questions have been answered to your satisfaction, or until you have been directed toward a better source of information.

PLANNING FOR GOOD NUTRITION

Every person with HIV has his or her individual nutritional needs—we cannot emphasize this enough! These needs vary according to a person's eating habits, medication schedule, energy needs, and nutritional status. That's why the first step should be to consult a registered dietitian who will help plan a diet that's right for you. Such a diet will have to provide enough calories, complex carbohydrates, protein, vitamins, and minerals to help your body fight the infection.

To help you meet these goals, or to help a caregiver assist you in meal planning, we provide a food guide designed specifically for people with HIV, along with recommendations based on that guide. You will notice that our guide is an inverted pyramid—not the standard food pyramid you may have seen before. We use the inverted pyramid for two reasons: one, to emphasize that the nutritional needs of a person with HIV are different than those of a person who is not infected, and two, to immediately draw your attention to the nutrients that are most important, starting with fluids and complex carbohydrates. To use this inverted pyramid, start at the top, with fluids, and move downward, paying particular attention to the serving amounts for each level.

Knowing what types and amounts of foods to eat is important, but it is equally important that you know how to keep track of what you eat. For that reason, we also provide a food diary (page 17). In addition, it is essential that you keep track of your weight—remember that malnourishment is a common problem among people with HIV. Therefore, we provide a weight chart (page 24). And finally, since standard medicine does not yet have a definitive solution to the problem of HIV, we review nontraditional diets and health remedies.

Nutrition Recommendations: Using the Food Guide

It is easier to plan a balanced, nutritious diet if you know how much of what types of food should be included in each day's meals. To help you plan meals, a food guide (Figure 1) and table (Table 1) are provided. Although the guide and table were both developed with HIV-positive persons in mind, it is important to remember that individual needs will vary.

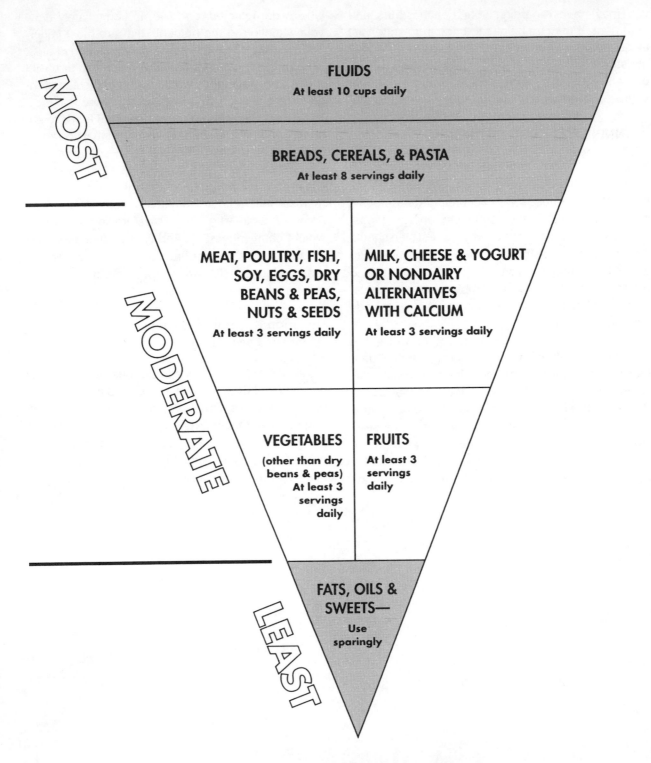

Figure 1. Food Guide for People Living with HIV

Table 1. Food Table for People Living With HIV

Food Group	Suggested Daily Servings	What Makes Up a Serving
Fluids	At least 10 cups—1 cup for every 15 pounds of body weight	1 cup low-fat milk, light soymilk, milk shake, nectar, fruit juice, vegetable juice, electrolyte drink (see page 38), water, broth, herbal tea, or blender drink (see page 109) Note: Nutrient-dense fluids will help meet calorie and protein goals. Water and tea may not be the best choices if you are trying to gain weight
Breads, Cereals, and Pastas	At least 8 servings	Choose whole-grain products: 1 slice of bread; half of a hamburger bun, bagel, or English muffin; a small roll, biscuit, muffin, or piece of corn bread; ½ cup cooked cereal, rice, or pasta; 1 small potato or half of a large potato; ¾ cup ready-to-eat breakfast cereal; 1 tortilla; half of a plantain; 6 plain crackers; 3 graham crackers
Meat, Poultry, Fish, Soy, Eggs, Dry Beans and Peas, Nuts, and Seeds	At least 3 servings	Choose lean cuts of meat and limit fried food: 3 ounces of cooked meat, fish, or poultry; 2 eggs; 4 tablespoons peanut butter; ¾ cup tofu; 1 cup cooked beans; ½ cup nuts Note: Half of a chicken breast is about 3 ounces, or 1 serving. A 3-ounce portion of meat is about the size and thickness of a deck of cards
Milk, Cheese, Yogurt, or Nondairy Alternatives With Calcium	At least 3 servings; 4 servings for women who are pregnant or breastfeeding, and for teens; 5 servings for teens who are pregnant or breastfeeding	Choose low-fat or nonfat dairy items: 1 cup milk, fortified soymilk, or lactose-reduced milk; 1 cup yogurt; 2 ounces cheese; ½ cup cottage cheese Note: Other rich sources of calcium include 3 ½ ounces sardines or salmon with bones, or 2 cups arugula, turnip greens, or dandelion greens
Fruits	At least 3 servings	A whole fruit, such as a medium-sized apple, banana, or orange; half a grapefruit; a wedge of melon; ¾ cup juice; ½ cup berries; ½ cup cooked or canned fruit; ¼ cup dried fruit Note: Choose fruits rich in vitamins A and C every day— see Table 2 (page 19). Wash all fruits thoroughly before eating
Vegetables	At least 3 servings	½ cup cooked vegetables; 1 cup chopped raw vegetables; 1 cup leafy raw vegetables such as spinach or lettuce; ¾ cup vegetable juice Note: Choose vegetables rich in vitamins A and C every day— see Table 2 (page 19). Wash all raw vegetables thoroughly before eating

Food Group	Suggested Daily Servings	What Makes Up a Serving
Fats, Sweets, and Oils	Foods from this group should be consumed sparingly if weight loss is not a problem. If weight loss is a problem, a moderate amount of fats, sweets, and oils can be added to the diet in addition to the recommendations made for the other food groups	Examples of fats and oils include: butter, margarine, shortening, lard, mayonnaise, cream sauces, avocado, olives, and olive oil Examples of sweets include: sugar, honey, jam, jelly, syrup, candy, gelatin, molasses, and most desserts

Fluid Recommendations

You should drink one cup of fluid for every fifteen pounds of body weight each day, or approximately ten glasses of fluid each day. Fluids and electrolytes—elements that allow the body to regulate electrical charges and control the flow of water into cells—provide the environment that supports the life of all the body's cells. The body's principle electrolytes are sodium, chloride, phosphorous, and potassium. Increase the amount of fluids consumed when fever, vomiting, or diarrhea are present, or if you are taking certain protease inhibitors (check with your health care professional), because these conditions can contribute to dehydration and electrolyte imbalances.

Plain water is not always the best choice. Fruit and vegetable juices and nectars, milk shakes, homemade blender drinks (see page 109), and electrolyte drinks (see page 38) can add calories and electrolytes.

Carbohydrate Recommendations

Complex carbohydrates are the source of many nutrients, and should make up the bulk of the calories you eat. They help provide and regulate the energy the body needs to rebuild and maintain lean body mass, and to fight fatigue.

Foods rich in complex carbohydrates should be eaten every two to three hours throughout the day. Good sources of complex carbohydrates include corn, potatoes, pasta, tortillas, rice, breakfast cereals, breads, kasha, and couscous.

On the other hand, you should limit simple carbohydrates, which provide calories but are usually low in nutrients. Refined sugars, such as table sugar, syrup, honey, and jellies, are simple carbohydrates.

Protein Recommendations

Eating an adequate amount of protein is essential for a person with HIV disease. Protein keeps the immune system strong and resistant to infection. It is also essential for the growth and repair of cells, and for the building of new tissue, including proper wound healing and the building of lean body mass. Protein requirements increase during times of stress, fever, and infection.

Lean proteins are your best choice. These include lean meats, poultry, eggs, fish, legumes such as peas and beans, low-fat milk, low-fat yogurt, cottage cheese, and low-fat cheeses.

Fat Recommendations

Excess fat is not healthy for anyone. Foods high in fat are often low in many other important nutrients. Also, high-fat foods can be difficult to digest, and can thus worsen symptoms such as nausea, vomiting, diarrhea, constipation, fatigue, and loss of appetite. Moreover, when a healthy individual goes without food for an extended length of time, the body will break down fat first to use as an energy source. However, research has shown that when the body is under stress, such as illness, fever, or infection, it relies more on protein than on fat as an energy source. A person with HIV should rely on foods high in protein and complex carbohydrates, rather than on fat, to provide the body with the energy it needs.

Monounsaturated fats, such as olive, peanut, and canola oils, are the best type of fats to use—in moderation, of course. You should limit your intake of saturated fats, such as shortenings and butter. Consumption of polyunsaturated fats, such as safflower, corn, and sesame oils, should also be limited because an excess intake of these oils may be associated with increased free-radical production—a process that places more stress on the immune system.

Fat consumption can be reduced by substituting skinless chicken, turkey, and fish for red meats, and by eliminating or reducing consumption of fried foods and goods baked with saturated fats. Bake, broil, grill, or stir-fry proteins, and avoid pan or deep-fat frying.

Read the labels on prepackaged, processed, and frozen foods. There are many foods on the market now that cater to consumers interested in low-fat diets. Just be sure that any low-fat claims are true by checking the type of oil used and the manner in which the foods are prepared. You should also be aware that many nonfat or low-fat baked goods have high sugar contents.

Vitamin and Mineral Recommendations

Vitamins and minerals play a critical role in the nutritional status of a person with HIV disease. Most vitamins and minerals affect immune function at some level, with some having more influence than others. Some research suggests that when vitamin and mineral deficiencies occur early in the course of HIV disease, the immune system may lose function faster and the disease may progress more quickly.

Generally, the best way to get the vitamins and minerals you need is to eat a wide variety of foods. Follow the food guide in Figure 1 for general daily diet recommendations. Fluids, at the top of the guide, provide the water and electrolytes the body needs every day. Breads, cereals, and pasta are excellent sources of most of the B vitamins, vitamin

E, zinc, and selenium. Meats, poultry, fish, soy, eggs, dry beans and peas, nuts, and seeds will provide you with good amounts of thiamin, riboflavin, niacin, B6, B12, folate, selenium, and zinc. Milk, cheese, and yogurt are good sources of vitamins A and D, and of calcium, riboflavin, and niacin. Vegetables and fruits are important sources of vitamin C, folate, and beta-carotene (which the body converts to vitamin A). Within the fats and oils, you can find sources of vitamins E and K. For the best specific food sources of the various vitamins and minerals, refer to Table 2.

In addition to a well-balanced meal plan, research does indicate that a daily supplement is a safe, inexpensive therapy that may offer good protection against AIDS in people already infected with HIV. There are no routinely prescribed vitamin and mineral dosages for HIV-infected individuals, because there have not been enough conclusive studies and each individual will have specific nutritional needs. A safe recommendation, however, is to take a multivitamin supplement with minerals that does not contain extra iron one to two times a day, one B-complex pill a day, 1 to 3 grams of vitamin C each day, and 400 to 800 International Units (IUs) of vitamin E each day.

Supplementation, in any amount, is an individual choice you should make with guidance from a health care professional. Keep in mind that vitamin and mineral supplements cannot replace a well-balanced, healthful diet. Always consult your health care professional or registered dietitian before increasing the dosage of any vitamin or mineral. (See Table 2 for specific information.)

Charting Your Course

What is your nutritional state right now? It is important to answer this question at the beginning of the planning process, and you can help find that answer by keeping a food diary and a weight chart.

Keeping a Food Diary

As someone with HIV, it is important that you keep track of what you're eating to help monitor weight, symptoms, and overall nutrition status. The best way to do that is to keep a food diary at the beginning of the planning process, and every three months (or as symptoms and weight changes dictate) afterwards. The three-day food diary in Worksheet 1 will help you and your dietitian evaluate your diet and identify your nutritional needs. To use the diary:

- Record everything you eat for a minimum of three consecutive days, including one day of a weekend and two days during the week, to get a complete picture of your eating habits and food choices. For instance, record your meals for a Thursday, Friday, and Saturday.

- Carefully estimate the quantity of foods and fluids consumed, including all meals, snacks, and beverages. Try to identify the ingredients in each dish.

- Make sure the amount of food you record reflects the amount after cooking. For instance, hamburger will shrink during cooking.

- Record the information within one hour after you've eaten to assure accuracy.

A sample diary is included as a guide.

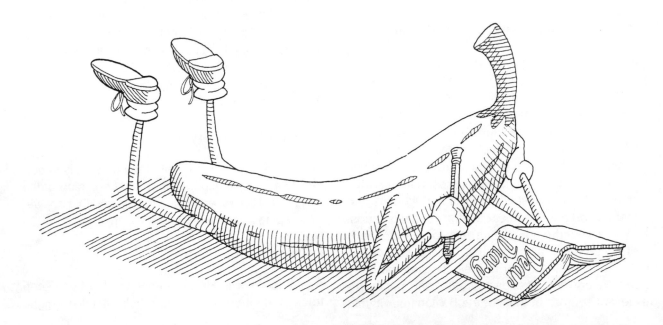

Table 2. Vitamin and Mineral Supplementation Recommendations

Vitamin/Mineral Function in the Body	Dietary Sources	RDA*	Safe Dosage Levels for HIV	Possible Harmful Levels
Vitamin A This fat-soluble vitamin is necessary for normal vision and for healthy cell structure. It helps keep skin healthy and protects against infection in the linings of the mouth, nose, throat, lungs, and digestive and urinary tracts	Liver, fortified milk, eggs, cheese, fish oil, fruits and vegetables that contain beta-carotene (see next entry)	10,000 IU** for men 8,000 IU** for women	Not recommended	Amounts greater than 25,000 IU** can prove toxic. Toxic levels can cause nerve damage, liver damage, headache, vomiting, loss of hair, and an unsteady gait
Beta-carotene This antioxidant is converted in the body to vitamin A as needed	Sweet potatoes, dark leafy vegetables, carrots, winter squash, red bell peppers, cantaloupes, tomatoes, apricots, mangoes, and peaches	No RDA	15 mg (25,000 IU**) for men and women	No known toxic level
Thiamin (B$_1$) This water-soluble vitamin helps the body break down and use carbohydrates. It is important for healthy nerves and muscles, and for normal heart function. A mild deficiency may cause loss of appetite, fatigue, irritability, and disturbed sleep. A deficiency may also cause night blindness, dry rough skin, loss of appetite, and diarrhea	Whole grain or enriched cereals and breads, brewer's yeast, pork, liver, brown rice, fish, peas, beans, nuts, eggs, and wheat germ	1.5 mg for men 1.1 mg for women	Up to 50 mg	No known toxic level. However, prolonged use of thiamin may deplete other B vitamins. Therefore, it should be taken in a B-complex form
Riboflavin (B$_2$) This water-soluble vitamin helps the body break down and use carbohydrates, fats, and proteins. It is needed for the body's use of other B-complex vitamins. A deficiency may cause a reduction in antibody production after immunization. A prolonged deficiency may also lead to chapped lips, cracks and sores in the corners of the mouth, a sore tongue, and sensitivity to light	Milk, cheese, yogurt, meat, fish, poultry, whole grain or enriched cereals and breads, dark leafy vegetables, liver, peas, beans, nuts, and eggs	1.7 mg for men 1.3 mg for women	Up to 50 mg	No known toxic level

Vitamin/Mineral Function in the Body	Dietary Sources	RDA*	Safe Dosage Levels for HIV	Possible Harmful Levels
Niacin (B$_3$) This water-soluble vitamin helps maintain the function of the skin, nerves, and gastrointestinal tract. It also aids in the release of energy from foods	Nuts, milk, cheese, yogurt, lean meats, poultry, fish, eggs, whole grain or enriched cereals and breads, peanut butter, and brewer's yeast	19 mg for men 15 mg for women	Up to 50 mg	Amounts equal to or greater than 1 gram have been reported to cause gastrointestinal distress, including nausea, vomiting, and diarrhea, and/or a burning sensation of the skin. Amounts greater than 3 grams can prove toxic. Toxic levels can cause rashes, liver damage, ulcers, skin flushes, and irregular heartbeat
Pyroxidine (B$_6$) This water-soluble vitamin plays an important role in maintaining the normal function of the immune system. It can help prevent anemia, skin lesions, and nerve damage. Deficiencies may result in a decrease in white blood cell count and antibody production, possibly reducing resistance to cancer and other diseases	Chicken, fish, pork, eggs, rice, peas, beans, soybeans, oats, whole wheat products, nuts, bananas, meat, and wheat germ	2.0 mg for men 1.6 mg for women	Up to 50 mg	Doses of 50 mg or more a day have been reported to cause numbness and tingling in the extremities. If these symptoms occur, reduce your dosage and consult your health care professional
Vitamin B$_{12}$ This water-soluble vitamin is essential for the manufacture of the genetic material in cells and, therefore, for growth and development. It also plays a role in the formation of red blood cells and helps prevent pernicious anemia. This vitamin helps the body use folic acid and carbohydrates, and helps maintain a healthy nervous system. A deficiency may cause a reduction in white blood cell function and impair the immune response, which can increase susceptibility to infection. A deficiency may also cause anemia, sore mouth and tongue, numbness and tingling of the limbs, memory loss, and depression	Liver, kidney, lean meats, fish, chicken, eggs, blue and green algae, milk, cheese, nutritional yeast, yogurt, whole grain or enriched cereals and breads, and fortified soy products. Note: plant foods do not contain vitamin B$_{12}$	2.0 mcg for men and women	Up to 100 mcg	No known toxic level

Vitamin/Mineral Function in the Body	Dietary Sources	RDA*	Safe Dosage Levels for HIV	Possible Harmful Levels
Folate (B-complex vitamin) This water-soluble vitamin is essential for growth and reproduction, and for the body's use of protein. It is important for the formation of red blood cells, and the development and proper function of the nervous system. A deficiency may cause a reduction in white blood cell count, which can increase susceptibility to infection. A deficiency may also cause anemia	Liver, yeast, leafy green vegetables, egg yolks, peas, beans, asparagus, whole grain or enriched cereals and breads, wheat germ, and citrus fruit and juice	200 mcg for men 180 mcg for women	Up to 400 mcg	No known toxic level
Pantothenic Acid (B-complex vitamin) This water-soluble vitamin is essential for the conversion of sugars and fats into energy, and for the body's use of other vitamins. It is needed for the proper function of the nervous system and adrenal glands, and for normal growth and development. A deficiency may cause a decrease in antibody production	Meat—especially liver, fish, and kidney, plus brewer's yeast, wheat germ, royal jelly, whole grain or enriched cereals and breads, peas, beans, milk, and eggs	No RDA. Experts recommend 4 to 7 mg	Up to 50 mg	No known toxic level. However, ingestion of more than 20 grams has been reported to result in diarrhea and water retention
Vitamin C This water-soluble, antioxidant vitamin is essential for healthy cell structure. It helps maintain normal connective tissue, promotes healthy teeth and gums, aids in iron absorption, and is needed for proper wound healing. A deficiency can cause a decrease in general resistance and antibody response, which can increase susceptibility to infection. A deficiency can also lead to anemia and the destruction of red blood cells	Citrus fruits, green and red peppers, broccoli, tomatoes, potatoes, cauliflower, arugula, persimmons, kiwis, papayas, cantaloupes, and strawberries	60 mg	1 to 3 grams	There is no known toxic level. However, doses over 1 gram may cause diarrhea, nausea, and stomach cramps. If these symptoms occur, consult your health care professional
Vitamin E This fat-soluble antioxidant vitamin helps in the formation of red blood cells and in the body's use of vitamin K. A deficiency can cause a decrease in general resistance and antibody response, which can increase susceptibility to infection. A deficiency can also lead to anemia and the destruction of red blood cells	Vegetable oils, wheat germ, nuts, green leafy vegetables, whole grain or enriched cereals and breads, seeds, olives, and asparagus	15 IU** for men 12 IU** for women	400 to 800 IU**	Doses of 1,200 IU** or more have reported to cause fatigue, high blood pressure, diarrhea, and headaches

Vitamin/Mineral Function in the Body	Dietary Sources	RDA*	Safe Dosage Levels for HIV	Possible Harmful Levels
Selenium This mineral is an antioxidant needed for proper immune response. It also improves the supply of oxygen to the heart muscle, thereby increasing endurance. A deficiency may cause impaired antibody production and may impair the killing of bacteria, which can lead to increased susceptibility to infection	Seafood, kidney, liver, eggs, grains, seeds, and garlic	70 mcg for men 55 mcg for women	50 to 150 mcg	Doses greater than 200 mcg per day may suppress immune cell function
Zinc This mineral is an antioxidant important for wound and burn healing, and is needed for the formation of proteins and nucleic acids. It helps the body use carbohydrates. A deficiency may cause a loss of appetite and affect the sense of taste. A severe deficiency may result in hair loss, rash, and inflammation of the mouth, tongue, eyelids, and areas around the fingernails	Dark-meat turkey, lamb, liver, tuna, eggs, seafood, whole grain breads and cereals, pumpkin seeds, sunflower seeds, and nuts	15 mg for men 12 mg for women	15 mg for men 12 mg for women	Amounts greater than 25 mg may cause stomach irritations and anemia, and may interfere with copper intake. Amounts greater than 100 mg may weaken immune response

*Recommended Dietary Allowances, published in 1989, are adequate and safe recommendations for the majority of healthy individuals who are neither pregnant nor breastfeeding. Always consult with your health care provider or registered dietitian to ensure adequate and safe intake.

**International Units.

Sources
1. National Research Council. Recommended Dietary Allowances. 10th Edition. Washington DC: Nation Academy Press, 1989.
2. The American Medical Association Guide to Prescription and Over-the-Counter Drugs. New York: Random House, 1988.
3. Bulletin of Experimental Treatments for AIDS. Nutritional Intervention in HIV disease. March 1994.

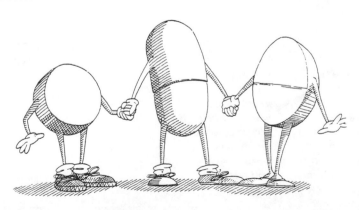

Worksheet 1. Three-Day Food Diary

DATE: **DAY OF THE WEEK:**

TIME	PLACE	AMOUNT	FOOD/BEVERAGE	PREP

Sample Diary

DATE: 1/10/95   **DAY OF THE WEEK: Thursday**

TIME	PLACE	AMOUNT	FOOD/BEVERAGE	PREP
12 noon	home	2 slices 2 ounces 1 tbsp 1 slice 1 1 cup	whole wheat bread lean ham mustard tomato fresh medium-sized apple milk	
3 pm	cafe	1 cup	low-fat berry yogurt	
6 pm	home	5 ounces 1 $\frac{1}{4}$ cup $\frac{1}{2}$ cup	skinless chicken potato low-fat sour cream mixed vegetables	broiled baked steamed

Keeping a Weight Chart

Maintaining weight is critical for someone with HIV because of the malnutrition and body wasting that often accompany HIV disease. Therefore, it is a good idea to keep a weight chart at the beginning of the planning process, or as symptoms and weight changes dictate. This will allow you to monitor your weight, and take steps to correct weight loss before other problems arise.

Worksheets 2 and 3 shows a weight chart and graph. Record your weight once a week on the same day and at the same time. Remember to wear the same amount of clothes each time. Also, use the same scale, since scales will vary.

If you start to lose weight, keep track of the foods you eat for a couple of days to see if this will help determine the cause of your weight loss (see the food diary in Figure 2). Determine if your eating habits have changed. Are you eating enough calories and nutrients? Are you experiencing any symptoms that may be contributing to your weight loss?

To use the chart and graph:

1. Record the first week's weight in the "Weight in Pounds" box for "Week 1" (Worksheet 2).

2. Record the second week's weight in the "Weight in Pounds" for "Week 2." Compare weight from week 2 to week 1.

3. Record the difference in weight (plus or minus pounds) from Week 1 in the Weight Change" box for Week 2.

4. Plot the weight change on the graph (Worksheet 3). Week 1's weight should appear as "0" on the grid, and weights for subsequent weeks will be plus or minus from "0."

5. Continue these steps for subsequent weeks, *always comparing the current week's weight to week 1.*

Reviewing Nontraditional Diets and Health Remedies

There are many products and dietary regimes on the

Worksheet 2. Weight Chart

Week	Date	Weight in pounds	Weight Change	Week	Date	Weight in pounds	Weight Change
1			X	27			
2				28			
3				29			
4				30			
5				31			
6				32			
7				33			
8				34			
9				35			
10				36			
11				37			
12				38			
13				39			
14				40			
15				41			
16				42			
17				43			
18				44			
19				45			
20				46			
21				47			
22				48			
23				49			
24				50			
25				51			
26				52			

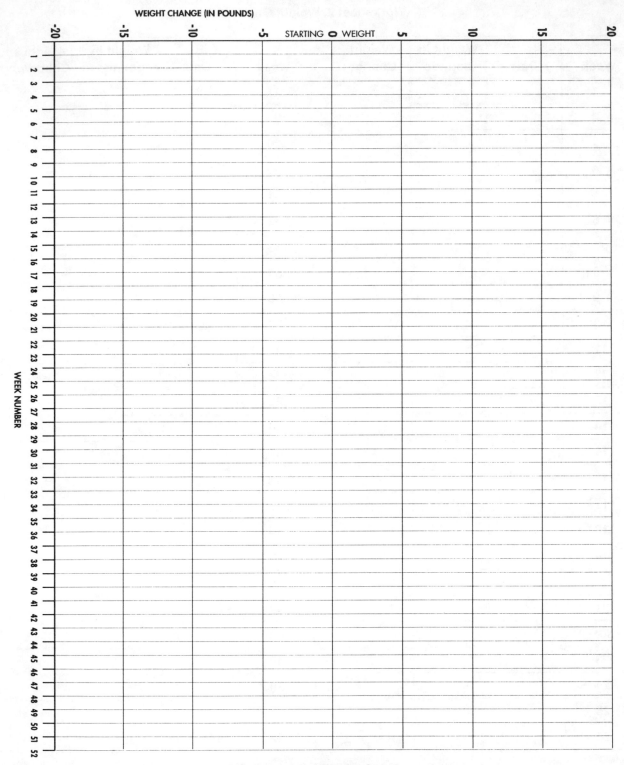

WEIGHT CHANGE (IN POUNDS)

Worksheet 3. Weight Graph

market that promise quick cures for HIV. These include teas, drinks, herbs, supplements, and alternative diets. Scientific journals do not cover many nontraditional diets or food products, so they may provide benefits as yet unknown by the scientific community.

A person with HIV who wants to try new products or diets should take the time to consult with his or her health care team, which can help evaluate any promised benefits. If a product doesn't produce harmful side effects, seems helpful, and is affordable, it may be worth a try.

Keep the following points in mind when considering the use of new, untested products:

- If it sounds too good to be true, it probably is.
- Watch out for words such as "amazing" or "miraculous." A responsible practitioner or scientist would probably not use these words.
- Don't be misled by a scientific-sounding explanation. Stop and determine what is really being promised. Ask your health care professional whether the explanation sounds valid or not.

DEVELOPING AN EXERCISE PROGRAM

A well-rounded fitness program plays an essential part in an HIV treatment plan. Regular exercise can build, maintain, and strengthen lean body mass; increase endurance and lung capacity; decrease stress; and improve sleeping patterns, appetite, and bowel movements. An exercise program should fit the individual's level of endurance, which means starting slowly for someone who is not used to physical exertion.

A complete fitness program should include both aerobic and anaerobic exercise. Aerobic exercise is any activity that leads to better use of oxygen within the body. This type of exercise improves heart and lung function, and strengthens the muscles, but usually does not increase lean body mass. Walking, swimming, jogging, cycling, and cross-country skiing are examples of aerobic exercise.

Anaerobic exercise requires less oxygen than aerobic exercise. Because anaerobic exercise helps build and maintain lean body mass, it is important for a person with HIV to include anaerobic exercise in his or her exercise routine. Weightlifting and push-ups are anaerobic exercises one can do at home. If fatigue is one of your symptoms, make anaerobic exercise your first priority.

Short periods of both aerobic and anaerobic exercise several times a week are better than one long period of exercise. Start slowly and build your endurance until you can comfortably exercise for at least twenty minutes at a time at least three times a week. Make sure to consult your health care professional before beginning any exercise program.

Working with a professional fitness trainer is an excellent way to help prevent injuries and improve technique, and to help plan a fitness routine that's right for you. There are trainers who specialize in working with individuals with HIV, trainers who are more aware of possible limitations in training and who know which exercises would be the most effective. To find such a specialist, contact your local AIDS or HIV organization.

Remember that the calories and fluids lost during exercise must be replaced. A small meal rich in carbohydrates should be eaten forty-five minutes before exercising, and within one hour after exercising, to replace calories. Fluids should be replaced by drinking electrolyte drinks (see page 38) or diluted juices.

The keys to a successful exercise program are to avoid overexertion or fatigue, and to exercise on a regular schedule.

REDUCING AND CONTROLLING STRESS

Reducing and controlling stress is an important part of maintaining overall health. The emotional stress of living with a chronic illness can greatly add to the physical stress, robbing you of both physical and emotional well-being. Depression, stress, and anxiety can all lead to poor eating habits, lack of sleep and, consequently, poor physical health.

Often, people are unwilling or unable to ask for help. Give yourself permission to accept emotional support from others just as you would accept medical treatment. Consider seeking professional guidance to help you better cope with this added stress. You may not always want or need emotional support

Changing Unhealthy Habits

People with HIV should avoid using tobacco, caffeine, alcohol, and recreational drugs. These substances can further weaken an already suppressed immune system, interfere with appetite, and contribute to malnutrition and weight loss. It is especially critical to avoid alcohol if you are taking a protease inhibitor (check with your health care professional), as both these substances place additional stress on the liver.

You may find that cutting down on the use of these substances is difficult, but there are ways to make the process easier. There are many smoking-cessation aids and programs on the market, and books such as *No If's, And's, or Butts*. There are cereal-based coffees, plus a wide variety of decaffeinated coffees. There is also an ever-widening array of decaffeinated teas, including a large selection of herbal teas. And there are nonalcoholic beers, and even some nonalcoholic wines, on the market.

If you are addicted to either alcohol or drugs, you will probably need help in overcoming your addiction. Your health care professional can help you find a treatment program.

from a professional, but take the time to find out what help is available, and take advantage of this help when appropriate.

Track your emotional well-being as you would your physical condition. Pay attention to your moods and to the stressful situations that take place in your daily life. Make a conscious effort to limit or avoid stress and to take care of your emotional state. Take the time for both play and rest.

If stress is a factor in your life, consult a competent licensed counselor in the HIV community and join an HIV support group in your area (see the Resource List). You also may want to explore such stress-reduction methods as meditation, biofeedback, visualization, or yoga. Establish a support network of friends and family who understand you and will give you the support you need. Stick with what works for you.

PRACTICING FOOD AND WATER SAFETY

It is crucial that a person with HIV disease practice the safe handling and preparation of food, and monitor the safety of the water supply. If this isn't done, food- or water-borne diseases and the symptoms they cause can further weaken the immune system, hastening the progression of HIV disease. Food- or water-borne illness can even prove fatal.

Symptoms of food- or water-borne illness include nausea, vomiting, diarrhea, cramping, and headache. Bacteria in the intestinal tract will cause symptoms to appear in approximately twelve to thirty-six hours, and may last from two to three days to several weeks. Toxins produced by bacteria will most likely cause symptoms to appear more rapidly—possibly as quickly as one to six hours after eating.

There are numerous conditions that can cause food- or water-borne illness, including:

- Exposing food to dirt or filth
- Handling food with dirty hands, or not washing one's hands after using the bathroom
- Cooking or preparing food with dirty equipment
- Failing to cook food to the correct temperature and for the proper length of time
- Failing to refrigerate fresh or cooked food
- Cooking with contaminated water without reaching a safe boil
- Drinking contaminated water
- Washing foods in contaminated water
- Brushing one's teeth with contaminated water
- Preparing noncooked recipes or drinks with contaminated water

There are ways to greatly reduce the risk of contracting a food- or water-borne illness. These safety rules cover shopping, storage, and preparation, as well as foods that should be avoided. Keep in mind that you cannot always detect contaminated food and the germs that cause food-borne illness through taste, touch, smell, or appearance.

Shopping Safety

The concern for food safety starts in the grocery store. When shopping:

- Organize the grocery list before going out. Pick up nonperishable items before perishable items. Pick up dairy products, meat, and frozen foods last, and refrigerate or freeze them as soon as possible. Never leave food in a hot car!
- Make sure that frozen foods are solid, and that refrigerated foods are cold.
- While shopping, put meats in plastic bags so that blood will not drip on other foods. Discard foods contaminated with blood from other products.
- Check the "sell-by" and "expiration" dates on product labels to make sure products are still safe.
- Don't buy cans that are dented, swollen, or damaged, or items with broken safety seals.

Storage Safety

Once the food is bought safely, it must be stored safely. When storing foods:

- Keep cold foods cold. Keep your refrigerator temperature below 40°F.
- Refrigerate all dairy products, including milk, eggs, and cheese.
- Make sure your freezer temperature is set at 0°F.
- Keep hot foods hot—above 140°F—until you're ready to eat or store them.
- Refrigerate or freeze leftovers immediately. To cool leftovers quickly, transfer large amounts into smaller containers.

Table 3. The Storage Life of Cold Food

Food	Refrigerator Life	Freezer Life
Cheese	2 to 4 weeks	9 months
Cottage cheese	2 to 3 days after opening	Don't freeze
Fish, raw	1 to 2 days	3 to 6 months
Eggs, uncooked in shell	3 weeks	Don't freeze
Raw egg yolks or whites, out of shell	2 to 4 days	Don't freeze
Eggs, hard-boiled	1 week	Don't freeze
Ground hamburger, pork, turkey, or lamb	1 to 2 days	3 to 4 months
Hot dogs	1 week	9 months
Leftovers (cooked meat)	2 to 3 days	2 to 3 months
Luncheon meats	4 to 7 days	1 to 2 months
Margarine/butter	1 to 2 weeks	4 to 6 months
Mayonnaise	2 months	Don't freeze
Meats, raw	2 to 3 days	4 to 6 months
Milk	5 days past carton date	Don't freeze
Poultry, raw	1 to 2 days	4 to 6 months
Poultry, cooked	2 to 3 days	2 to 3 months
Salads	Up to 3 days	Don't freeze
Soups or stews	2 to 3 days	2 to 3 months
TV dinners	Store frozen	3 to 4 months

NOTE: Store all meats in freezer wrap.

- Label and date all leftovers, and periodically check the expiration date on all foods you store. Know how long foods will stay safe in the refrigerator or freezer, and dispose of foods that are past the date specified (see Table 3).
- Store raw and cooked foods in separate sections of your refrigerator. Put raw foods in double bags and store on the bottom shelf to avoid having their juices drip onto other foods.
- Do not wash berries, cherries, and plums before refrigeration, since moisture increases the likelihood that mold will grow.
- Store dry and canned goods in a cool, dry place. The optimum storage temperature is

50°F to 70°F. It's important to remember that canned goods are subject to spoilage and deterioration in quality over long periods of time. Acidic foods such as tomatoes and berries keep for a shorter period of time than nonacidic foods. Always wipe canned goods with a clean cloth before opening.

- Throw away cans with rust, bulges, leaks, or dents.

Preparation Safety

Efforts to safely buy and store food will be for nothing unless care is taken in the areas of cleanliness and food preparation. Keep the following cleanliness tips in mind:

- Wash hands frequently and carefully with an antibacterial soap and hot water, and remember to clean underneath your fingernails, which should be kept short. Keep disinfectant hand soap near the kitchen sink to encourage frequent washing. You should wash your hands after using the bathroom, handling garbage or pets, touching dirty dishes, smoking, coughing, scratching skin or hair, or handling raw food, and before beginning food preparation.

- Clean and disinfect work surfaces, cutting boards, dishtowels, sponges, and utensils frequently to avoid cross-contamination of bacteria from raw foods to cooked foods. Sanitize with a solution made of ten parts water to one part bleach. Rinse items thoroughly before you use them.

- To further avoid cross-contamination, always disinfect surfaces and utensils that have come in contact with raw meat or poultry before you use them to serve cooked food.

When preparing food:

- Don't thaw foods at room temperature. Thaw frozen meats, fish, egg products, and poultry in the refrigerator or microwave. Never refreeze thawed meat products.

- Always make sure that eggs are cooked until well

Table 4. Safe Cooking Temperatures

Type of Food	Temperature*
Meats	to 165°F or higher
Poultry	to 180°F
Eggs	160°F
Homemade soups and stews	170°F

*Note: To be certain of temperatures, use a meat thermometer.

done because they can carry salmonella, a bacteria that causes food poisoning.

- Cook meat, poultry, and fish until well done and the juices run clear (see Table 4 for correct temperatures). To be certain of temperatures, use a meat thermometer.

- Use only pasteurized milk and dairy products.

- Wash raw fruits and vegetables thoroughly before you eat or cook them. Use one tablespoon of bleach to one gallon of water or twenty drops of 2 percent iodine tincture to one gallon of water—iodine tablets or tincture can be found in the pharmacy section of most grocery stores, or where camping supplies are sold. Let the iodine solution stand for ten minutes, then wash produce in the solution. Rinse well with water. Iodine may discolor food, but is harmless. Peeling fruits and vegetables will help eliminate some risk of contamination, but you should still rinse produce before peeling.

- Have more than one cutting board on hand: use one for raw meats, poultry, and fish; one for raw fruits and vegetables; and one for cooked meats. Always thoroughly wash cutting boards directly before and after use.

- Avoid tasting foods while cooking. Germs from your mouth can make foods spoil faster.

- Heat leftover foods thoroughly to an internal temperature of 165°F to 180°F (see Table 4). Use a meat thermometer for accuracy.

- Throw out all foods, including cheese, that show any sign of mold.

- Never taste or smell foods you suspect may be unsafe. You may eat or inhale harmful molds.
- When in doubt, throw it out!

Foods To Avoid

The following foods are easily contaminated and should be avoided:

- Raw or undercooked meat, poultry or fish, including sushi, sashimi, steak tartar, carpaccio, raw oysters, and ceviche
- Raw or soft-cooked eggs, and batters or recipes that contain raw eggs, including: raw cookie dough; poached or soft-boiled eggs; fried eggs with runny yolks; salad dressing made with raw eggs, such as caesar salad; milk shakes; hollandaise sauce; homemade ice cream; homemade mayonnaise; soft custard; and eggnog or blender drinks to which raw eggs have been added. A safe substitute for raw eggs is a pasteurized egg product or substitute
- Unwashed, raw produce
- Moldy fruit and vegetables, or produce that has soft spots or bruises
- Moldy bread or cheese—throw away the whole loaf or brick of cheese because mold spores can penetrate past the section where they are visible
- Cheeses made with mold, such as blue and Roquefort, especially if you have a low T cell count
- Soft-ripened cheeses, such as Brie and Camembert
- Unpasteurized milk and dairy products
- Refrigerated foods that have been left out at room temperature for longer than one hour
- Home-canned or smoked products, since there is a greater risk these foods may have been prepared improperly
- Perishable foods or liquids past their expiration date

And remember—when eating out, be assertive!

Ask about food freshness and preparation methods. Ask that meat, fish, and poultry be cooked until well done. Avoid salad bars because you cannot be sure whether or not the fruits and vegetables have been properly prepared and handled. Avoid restaurants in which the person handling the money is also preparing the food.

Check the Water Supply

Although tap water is generally safe, it can be contaminated with microorganisms such as cryptosporidia and giardia. To error on the side of caution, we recommend that all HIV-positive persons boil, filter, or buy their water. This is especially important if your T-cell count is low, or if you suspect your water is contaminated, or if you are traveling and are not sure about the source of the drinking water. To find out about your local water supply, contact your local water supplier—the phone number should be on your water bill—or the EPA Safe Drinking Hotline at 1-800-426-4791. To ensure that your water is safe:

- Boil the water. It's safe to drink water that has been at a rolling boil for one minute at sea level and three minutes when at an elevation above 6,500 feet.
- Filter the water. Make sure any filter you use removes particles smaller than one micron, or it may not catch the cryptosporidia parasites. You should replace the filter as directed. Also, make sure the filter has been tested and certified by the National Sanitation Foundation (NSF), and meets NSF standard number 53. Call the NSF at 1-800-673-8010 to find out which filter systems are certified.
- Buy distilled water. Distilled water meets the safety requirements for individuals with HIV.
- Buy mineral or spring water that is bottled by companies who are members of the International Bottled Water Association. This association has standards that meet the water safety requirements for persons living with HIV. To check the quality of a bottled water, either call the bottling company or the association at 1-800-WATER-11.

Don't forget to boil or filter *all* the water you consume, including water used in uncooked recipes and that used to make ice cubes, to make juice, to wash fruits and vegetables, and to brush your teeth.

THE COMPLETE APPROACH TO HEALTH MANAGEMENT

Remember, as the person who is living with HIV, you are the most important member of your health care team. Whether you have symptoms or not, your goals should be to:

- Build a team of health care professionals to help you develop a sound treatment plan
- Drink nutritious fluids often throughout the day
- Consume a diet high in complex carbohydrates and lean proteins as part of well-balanced meals that allow you to meet your individual nutrition and weight requirements
- Supplement your diet daily with a multivitamin with minerals, and discuss additional vitamin and mineral needs with your health care provider or dietitian
- Maintain a healthy body weight. Monitor your weight weekly—we recommend maintaining weight at 5 to 10 percent above your usual body weight. Remember, it's important to add pounds in the form of lean muscle rather than fat (see page 45 for specific weight-gain tips)
- Keep a food diary when appropriate
- Review nontraditional diets and food plans for effectiveness
- Limit or avoid harmful substances such as caffeine, alcohol, recreational drugs, and tobacco
- Exercise at a rate and frequency approved and monitored by your health care provider
- Limit stress and practice stress reduction methods
- Follow food and water safety rules to prevent or minimize your risk of food- or water-borne illness

Taking an active role in planning and managing your health—in partnership with your health care team—will help ensure that your treatment plan is truly designed to meet your specific needs. Remember, it may not be necessary to make broad lifestyle changes all at once. Work with your team to prioritize goals and design a plan that you will follow to make HIV infection a manageable, chronic disease. Setting realistic goals and planning for good nutrition will help you improve your quality of life.

Using Diet to Help Alleviate HIV Symptoms

During the course of HIV disease, many persons experience a wide range of symptoms due to opportunistic infections, medication side effects, unbalanced diets, food intolerances, stress, depression, and cancers associated with HIV disease. These symptoms can profoundly and negatively affect a person's interest in eating and ability to eat, and, therefore, can contribute to malnutrition and body wasting. Medications, when appropriate, should be used to treat any opportunistic infections that may be causing symptoms, but a well-designed nutritional strategy is also an important part of helping you feel better.

The most common symptoms associated with HIV disease are chewing and swallowing difficulties, dry mouth, mouth and throat sores, alterations in taste, loss of appetite, constipation, diarrhea, fatigue, and nausea and vomiting. In addition, it is important to fight body wasting by trying to add lean body mass.

COPING WITH COMMON SYMPTOMS

In this section, we help you cope with these symptoms by providing practical tips for living with each symptom, plus a complete one-week meal plan designed to help alleviate that symptom. The meal plans—which include three meals and three snacks a day—are all at the end of the section, and use some of the recipes contained in Part Two. They also specify what fluids should be drunk at each meal. Note that when we specify fruit nectar, we do mean something like peach nectar, which is a bit more substantial than plain fruit juice. You should consult with a dietitian to build similar meal plans for each week, using the recipe-by-symptoms charts at the beginning of each Part Two section to cross-reference symptoms with the recipes in this book.

If you are experiencing more than one symptom, make sure you cross-reference the tips offered in each section, and note any conflicting advice. If the advice conflicts, *follow all the "avoid" advice.* For instance, you may be experiencing both nausea and vomiting—for which you are advised to *try* citrus fruits or candies to soothe symptoms—and mouth sores—for which you are advised to *avoid* citrus fruits or candies. In this case, you would follow the "avoid" advice in order to not worsen your mouth sores. You would also follow other advice for both symptoms that does not conflict.

Dealing With Chewing and Swallowing Difficulties, Dry Mouth, and Mouth and Throat Sores

The lining of the mouth and throat is a sensitive area. Many people with HIV develop a soreness of or lesions on the gums, mouth, tongue, and throat; difficulty in chewing food due to irritation from infections such as candidiasis (thrush), dental complications, malnutrition, or medications; or dry mouth. Dysphagia—the inability to swallow normally—may also be a problem.

What follows are lists of ideas and a meal plan (page 48) to help make living with these symptoms a little easier. Also see "Practicing Good Oral Hygiene."

The following tips can help you adapt to chewing and swallowing difficulties:

- Eat soft-textured, moist foods, such as oatmeal, grits, canned fruits, cottage cheese, yogurt, mashed potatoes, noodles, soups, casseroles, soft milk shakes, creamed cereals, macaroni and cheese, pudding, custard, ice cream, applesauce, tofu, and all types of eggs, including mashed hard-boiled eggs.
- Purée foods in a blender when necessary. Experiment with the consistency to meet your taste and comfort needs. Add juice, milk, gravy, or stock to alter the consistency of puréed foods.
- Add moisture to dry foods with gravies, cream sauces, salad dressings, stock, sour cream, mayonnaise, butter, margarine, yogurt, milk, or soymilk. If fat absorption is a problem, remember to use low-fat or nonfat products.
- Drink liquids high in calories and protein, such as enriched blender drinks (see page 109), fortified milk (see page 115), fruit smoothies, and shakes.
- Avoid rough or course foods, such as breadsticks, toast, popcorn, dry granola bars, nuts, potato chips, dry cereals, and pretzels.
- Tilt your head either backward or forward to make swallowing easier.

The following tips can help you alleviate dry mouth:

- Add moisture to dry foods with gravies, cream sauces, salad dressings, stock, sour cream, mayonnaise, butter, margarine, yogurt, milk, or soymilk. If fat absorption is a problem, remember to use low-fat or nonfat products.
- Sip fluids throughout the day, such as fruit juices and nectars, and homemade blender drinks (see page 109).
- Stimulate the flow of saliva with sour candy, lemon wedges, chewing gum, or ice chips made from frozen juices.
- Avoid coffee and alcohol, which act as diuretics and may possibly cause dehydration.
- Ask your health care professional about artificial saliva or medications that can alleviate dry mouth.

The following tips can help you deal with mouth and throat sores:

- Avoid citrus or carbonated beverages, such as citrus fruit juices (orange, pineapple, lemon, or grapefruit), tomato juice, and soda.
- Avoid citrus fruits and acidic, spicy, and salty foods, such as oranges, pineapples, grapefruit, potato chips, chili, vinegar, red pepper, black pepper, and tomato sauce.
- Avoid hot foods. Cold or room temperature foods are generally less irritating.
- Avoid smoking cigarettes, using commercial mouthwash, and drinking alcohol.
- Try cold foods to help soothe your mouth and throat. Try sherbet, fruit ices, frozen yogurt, milk shakes, or ice cream.
- Avoid rough or course foods, such as breadsticks, toast, popcorn, dry granola bars, nuts, potato chips, dry cereals, and pretzels.
- Use straws cut in half to sip drinks or cooled soups. This will help fluid bypass sensitive areas in the mouth and reduce the amount of sucking required for ingestion.
- Drink soups or stock from a glass or cup, instead of using a spoon and bowl.

Practicing Good Oral Hygiene

Good oral hygiene is important for maintaining the health of your teeth and gums. In addition to getting good professional dental care, you should also practice good oral hygiene at home:

- At least three times a day, use a toothbrush with soft bristles (or a cotton swab) and a flavored toothpaste to clean your teeth, tongue, and gums.

- After you eat, rinse your mouth with a mixture of one cup of hydrogen peroxide to one cup of warm water. Swish the mixture around your mouth and then spit it out—don't swallow! If you are experiencing mouth and throat sores, you may want to dilute this mixture to avoid irritating the sores.
- If oral or esophageal thrush is a problem, remember to take your antifungal medication regularly.

Adapting To Alterations In Taste

People with HIV can also experience alterations in taste, such as a metallic taste experienced when eating meat. What follows are a list of ideas and a meal plan (page 50) to help make living with this symptom a little easier. Also read "Practicing Good Oral Hygiene."

The following tips can help you deal with alterations in taste:

- If your mouth is not sore, try swishing a small amount of ginger ale around in your mouth before eating to clear your palate.
- Try tart foods to help mask metallic tastes. If mouth sores are not present, add vinegar, lemon juice, pickles, or relish to your food. Drink lemonade or orange, cranberry, lemon, or pineapple juice. You also can try sucking on a slice of lemon or orange, or on sour candies before you eat.
- Try eating protein foods, such as chicken or beef, at a cold temperature, which may help lessen the aftertaste.
- If red meat doesn't taste right or leaves a metallic taste in your mouth, eat protein from other sources. Try chicken, turkey, or fish instead. You can also try eggs, dairy products, peanut butter, tofu, or cooked dry beans as protein substitutes.
- Eat foods that have been marinated to increase or alter flavors. Marinate meat, chicken, turkey, fish, or tofu in vinegar, sweet wine, salad dressing, sweet and sour sauce, fruit juices, or soy sauce.
- Add bacon bits, ham strips, sliced almonds, chopped onions, or cheese sauces to vegetables for more flavor.
- Use more seasonings with stronger flavors when you cook. Add fresh or dry herbs to your food, such as rosemary, thyme, basil, oregano, cumin, lemon juice, mint, cinnamon, nutmeg, and pepper.
- Choose foods that smell appealing.
- Try using plastic utensils instead of silverware. Plastic helps decrease the metallic taste for some people.
- Check with your health care professional about your possible need for a zinc supplement. Your body requires zinc for proper taste sensations. Don't add zinc to your diet unless you first consult your health care professional, since excess zinc can suppress the immune system.

Improving Appetite

Loss of appetite, also called anorexia, is a common symptom in HIV disease. Depression, stress, medication, fever, and pain can all affect appetite. You may not go through the same cycles of hunger as you did before. And without an appetite, it may become difficult to motivate yourself to eat.

How do you fight loss of appetite? The most important thing is to *not* wait for hunger to let you know when to eat. Remember, without nourishment the body—and especially the immune system—will not perform as well. Food provides the fuel to fight off infection. Think of eating as part of treatment. What follows are a list of ideas and a meal plan (page 52) to help make living with loss of appetite a little easier.

The following tips can help you improve appetite and integrate food back into your life:

- Make the commitment to eat! Talk with a dietitian, friends, or family members—people who will help motivate you and provide a support system.
- Eat by the clock. Because your body may not be giving you hunger signals, you need to place yourself on a schedule, as you would with medication. Try to eat or drink every two hours. Also, start with small portions. Larger meals may be overwhelming and may discourage you from eating.
- Eat foods high in protein and calories, so that you take in as many nutrients as possible at every meal. Try cheese and crackers, a peanut butter and banana sandwich, cereal and milk, a turkey sandwich, pizza, or a burrito.
- Avoid eating large amounts of fruits and vegetables, which are high in nutrients but low in calories.
- Drink calorie- and nutrient-dense beverages throughout the day. Good choices include fruit juices and nectars, fortified milk (see page 115) or milk alternatives, and homemade blender drinks (see page 109).
- Avoid consuming empty calories that may fill you

up but won't provide the nutrients your body needs. Examples of empty calories include water, coffee, soda, tea, stock, and gelatin, and junk foods such as chips or sweets.

- Keep snacks in easy-to-reach places, such as next to your favorite chair or near your bed. Make sure these are foods that remain safe at room temperature. Examples include crackers, dried fruit, nuts, pretzels, and trail mix (see page 136). Easy-to-reach snacks may encourage mindless snacking.
- Take advantage of any and all cravings or desires to eat. If you feel like eating a taco at 7 A.M.—go for it!
- Eat bigger snacks at bedtime. A big snack in the evening will be digested as you sleep, but eating a big snack earlier in the day may prevent you from eating other meals.
- Tempt your taste buds with your favorite foods, unless you're feeling nauseated. Avoid your favorite foods when nauseated because you don't want to start associating these foods with feeling ill.
- Talk with your health care professional about possible causes of your loss of appetite. Are you depressed, under stress, or in pain? Do you need to decrease or switch your medications?
- If your physical condition allows, take a walk for ten to fifteen minutes before eating. Mild exercise can stimulate the appetite.
- Make meal and snack time a pleasurable experience. Play your favorite music and place flowers on the table. Try adding colorful foods and seasonings to your meal, and cook foods with different textures.
- Avoid tobacco, alcohol, and other recreational drugs because these substances may suppress appetite.
- Speak to your health care professional about medications that may help stimulate your appetite.

Controlling Constipation

A lack of dietary fiber, intestinal complications, low liquid intake, emotional stress, lack of exercise, and some medications—particularly pain medications—can all contribute to constipation. Constipation is defined as a decrease in the frequency of bowel movements, accompanied by prolonged or difficult passage of stools.

The first step in addressing this symptom is a visit to your health care professional, to rule out the possibility of intestinal disease or other serious condition. Also, let your health care professional know about any medications you are taking, including antidepressants, antacids containing aluminum or calcium, pain medications such as codeine, antihistamines, or large quantities of laxatives. These can all contribute to constipation.

The next step is to review your diet. Poor diet can be a major contributor to constipation. Generally, you will want to increase intake of dietary fiber and liquid. Fiber is found in foods from the bread and cereal, vegetable, and fruit groups. To avoid disrupting the digestive system and increasing gas, it's a good idea to add high-fiber foods gradually.

What follows are a list of ideas and a meal plan (page 54) to help make living with constipation a little easier.

The following tips can help you control constipation:

- Eat more whole grains, such as kasha, brown rice, barley, and bulgur. Choose whole grain breads and cereals instead of refined products. For example, eat whole wheat or multigrain breads instead of white; all-bran cereal, granola, or oatmeal instead of high-sugar cereals; and bran or nut muffins instead of doughnuts or pastries. Add small amounts of wheat or oat bran to meals. For example, stir bran into yogurt, sprinkle it over cereal or eggs, or add it to pancake recipes.

- Eat at least the minimum servings of fruits and vegetables as recommended in the food guide on page 14. You can also try dried fruits, such as prunes, figs, and raisins.

- Eat more whole nuts, and seeds. Also eat more legumes, including lentils, split or black-eyed peas, and whole dried beans such as black, pinto, and kidney.

- Increase your fluid intake. Drink a minimum of one cup of fluid for every fifteen pounds of body weight. If you're trying to gain weight, water may not be the best choice because it does not contain any calories. Try fruit juices or nectars (particularly prune) and homemade blender drinks (see page 109) instead of water.

- Try warm or hot liquids, especially in the morning and evening. This may help stimulate bowel movement.

- Learn to relax. Stress can cause or aggravate constipation. Find soothing, pleasant activities that help you unwind. Try listening to music, watching your favorite television program, meditating, or spending time with people whose company you enjoy.

- Take time to exercise. Even moderate exercise can help combat constipation by moving food through the bowel faster. Walking is one of the best forms of exercise for this purpose.

- Avoid the overuse of chemical laxatives. Commercial chemical laxatives may provide relief initially, but often become addicting and can actually cause your constipation to become worse. If your health care professional suggests using laxatives, ask about natural or vegetable laxatives that contain crushed psyllium seed. Natural stool softeners are not addictive and are generally safe, even when taken over long periods.

Decreasing Diarrhea

Diarrhea is a problem for most people with HIV disease at some time during the course of their illness. Diarrhea is defined as the passage of frequent stools of a soft or liquid consistency. Chronic diarrhea is usually defined as the passage of three or more loose, watery stools a day for more than a month.

Diarrhea can cause the body to lose fluids, important electrolytes such as sodium and potassium, and nutrients. These losses may in turn lead to dehydration, electrolyte imbalances, body wasting, and malnutrition.

The first step in evaluating your approach to treatment should be to have a physical examination, including a review of your medical history. Let your health care professional know what you have been eating and drinking, including medications and vitamin supplements, and if you've been travelling recently.

Diarrhea may result from opportunistic infections associated with the disease, such as cryptosporidium, mycobacterium avium complex (MAC), or cytomegalovirus; diet, such as intolerance to foods containing lactose, caffeine, or fat; side effects from medications; megadoses of vitamin C; foodborne or water-borne illness; changes in the intestinal lining; or stress.

Even if the diarrhea can't be eliminated, a change in diet may help reduce its occurrence. The goal is to eat foods that provide important nutrients while eliminating or reducing foods that may be the cause of, or may aggravate, the diarrhea. Remember, foods that may cause problems for some people may not for others.

What follows are a list of ideas and a meal plan (page 56) to help make living with diarrhea a little easier. There's also information on how to deal with two common causes of diarrhea—fat malabsorption and lactose intolerance.

The following tips can help you reduce the occurrence of diarrhea:

- Increase the soluble fiber in your diet. Soluble fiber—fiber that dissolves in water—is binding and will slow the passage of food through your system. Soluble fiber is recommended in cases of diarrhea because its sponge-like consistency helps the intestines form stools by soaking up water. Foods high in soluble fiber include apples, apricots, pears, peaches, melons, strawberries, bananas, pearled barley, white rice, peas, beans, oat bran, and oatmeal. Also, try a product that contains crushed psyllium seed to help your intestines form stool and thus relieve your diarrhea.

Homemade Electrolyte Drink

Yield: 1 serving
Preparation time: 1 minute

2 cups water

1 to 1 1/2 cups infant rice
  cereal

1/2 teaspoon salt

Replenish fluids lost because of symptoms or exercise with this healthy, easy-to-prepare drink. If the consistency is too thick for your tastes, add more water.

1. Combine all ingredients. Stir, and serve immediately.

NUTRITION INFORMATION (PER SERVING):
Calories: 225   Fat: 2 g   Carbohydrates: 45 g   Protein: 5 g

- Decrease the insoluble fiber in your diet. Insoluble fiber—fiber that doesn't dissolve in water—can cause foods to move faster through your system. Foods high in insoluble fiber include corn, dried fruits, raw fruits and vegetables (except those listed under soluble fiber), nuts, seeds, popcorn, wheat bran and whole grain breads, and cereals (except oatmeal). Cook all vegetables to make them easier to digest.

- Decrease the level of fat in your diet, since your gastrointestinal tract may not fully digest or absorb it (see page 40).

- Decrease or avoid foods high in lactose—the sugar found in milk and dairy products—until you determine its effect on your system. Many individuals are unable to digest or absorb lactose, which results in diarrhea, gas, and bloating (see page 40).

- Talk with your health care professional about products that will help replenish the beneficial microorganisms that live in your intestines, especially if you are taking antibiotics. These microorganisms help you digest your food, and antibiotics often harm them.

- Avoid tobacco, alcohol, and foods containing caffeine, including coffee, tea, soda, and chocolate. These are gastrointestinal stimulants and can irritate your digestive system.

- Eat small meals frequently throughout the day to prevent stomach distention.

- Avoid foods that have a laxative effect, such as prunes, prune juice, and foods containing sorbitol, a sweetening agent found in sugar-free products.

- If you're experiencing cramping, bloating, or gas, avoid foods that may increase these symptoms. Avoid beans, foods containing sorbitol, carbonated drinks, cabbage, cauliflower, Brussels sprouts, broccoli, garlic, onions, and spicy foods.

- Try drinking most of your fluids between meals and snacks, instead of with meals.

- Decrease your stress levels, especially around mealtime. Stress may aggravate diarrhea. For example, increase your pleasure at mealtimes by eating in a relaxed atmosphere.

- Ask your health care professional about antidiarrheal or bulking medications. The medication will vary depending upon the cause of your diarrhea.

- Avoid foods prepared with olestra (trade-named Olean), an artificial fat that has been linked to diarrhea in studies.

Reducing the diarrhea itself is only part of the problem. It is also important to replenish lost nutrients and fluids:

- Drink plenty of fluids that are high in calories, protein, sodium, and potassium. Good fluid choices include homemade blender drinks (see page 109); stock; electrolyte drinks (see page 38); juices, such as diluted cranberry, grape, or apple juice; nectars, such as apricot, mango, peach, pear, or banana nectar; and vegetable juices. Drink a minimum of one cup of fluid for every fifteen pounds of your body weight. Your need for fluid will increase with the presence of fever, excessive sweating, and frequency of diarrhea and vomiting, and with the ingestion of protease inhibitors.

- Keep fluids within easy reach and sip them throughout the day.

- Eat foods high in potassium, which is an important electrolyte lost with the occurrence of diarrhea. Foods high in potassium include bananas, apricots, peaches, nectarines, potatoes, fish, tomatoes, and chicken.

- Try drinking fluids at room temperature. Hot or cold fluids may aggravate diarrhea.

- Remember to reintroduce the foods you enjoy eating, one at a time, after your symptoms have cleared or when you've determined that these foods don't aggravate your diarrhea.

Diarrhea Caused by Fat Malabsorption

Fat malabsorption is a condition in which fats are either poorly digested or not fully absorbed in the gastrointestinal tract. This condition often occurs when there is an infection in the intestinal tract. The presence of microorganisms such as cryptosporidium and mycobacterium avium complex (MAC) may impair the body's ability to digest fat. Decreased pancreatic or liver function may also cause fat malabsorption. You may want to discuss the benefits of pancreatic or digestive enzymes, supplements that can aid your body's ability to digest fats, with your health care professional.

Switch to a low-fat or nonfat diet and broil, bake, roast, or grill meat, fish, and poultry. Use egg whites for cooking instead of whole eggs. In addition, you may want to try cooking with a medium chain triglyceride (MCT) oil. This oil is easier for the body to absorb than most dietary fats and does not contribute to persistent diarrhea. However, MCT oil is fairly expensive.

Avoid foods high in fat, including:

- Deep-fried foods such as French fries, tempura, battered vegetables, and seafood
- Doughnuts and croissants
- Potato chips
- Bacon, sausage, ham, bologna, hot dogs, and pepperoni
- Tuna in oil
- Margarine, butter, and oil
- Whole milk and half-and-half
- Whole eggs and egg yolks
- Ice cream
- Mayonnaise
- Creamy salad dressings
- Cream sauces or gravies
- Olives
- Nuts and seeds
- Avocados

Switch to low-fat or nonfat foods, including:

- Nonfat milk or light soymilk
- Nonfat cottage cheese
- Nonfat yogurt
- Nonfat cream cheese
- Tuna packed in water
- Baked skinless chicken or turkey
- Fish
- Lean red meat—chuck or flank
- Canadian bacon
- Egg whites alone—two egg whites equal one whole egg
- Baked potatoes, white rice, pasta, or bread
- Fat-free condiments such as mustard, ketchup, or vinegar
- Angel food cake
- Bagels or pita bread
- Toast with honey or jam
- Whole beans, if gas is not a problem
- Sherbet, popsicles, gelatin, or ices
- Pretzels or breadsticks

Diarrhea Caused by Lactose Intolerance

Digestive discomfort after drinking milk or eating foods made with dairy products may indicate lactose intolerance. Lactose intolerance refers to the condition in which the body is unable to digest and absorb lactose—the sugar found in milk and dairy products. The cause of lactose intolerance is the absence of lactase, the enzyme responsible for breaking down lactose, in the system.

Lactose intolerance can be an inherited trait or linked to several gastrointestinal conditions, such as gastric surgery, chronic diarrhea, and intestinal infection. It can also be caused by certain medications, particularly antibiotics. It can be either a temporary or a permanent condition, depending upon the cause.

The most common symptoms of lactose intolerance are bloating, gas, cramping, and watery diarrhea. Symptoms may appear within fifteen to thirty minutes, or may take up to several hours to appear.

If you think you may be lactose intolerant, avoid foods and beverages that contain lactose for three to four days, while monitoring your symptoms. Also, check your medications to see if they contain lactose. If at the end of that time your symptoms have improved or cleared, this may indicate lactose was the cause of your symptoms and you may want to continue a lactose-free or low-lactose diet.

To avoid or limit foods high in lactose, it's important to read food labels and become familiar with foods that may contain lactose. Check the label for lactose, milk, nonfat milk, powder or dry milk, whey, casein, lactalbumin, sodium caseinate, butter, margarine, cheese, curds, sweet or sour cream, buttermilk, or malted milk.

Avoid these foods that are high in lactose:

- Milk products, including buttermilk and powdered, evaporated, and goat's milk
- Cheese, except that aged more than ninety days
- Butter and creams, including whipping cream, sour cream, and half-and-half
- Instant breakfast drinks
- Instant coffee
- Foods made with dairy products, such as pudding, custards, ice cream, salad dressings, cream sauces, and breads
- Cold cuts or frankfurters with added dry milk or milk solids

Try these foods that are low in lactose:

- Lactose-reduced milk, or lactase enzyme (in caplet or liquid form) that is added to dairy products before consumption

- Natural cheeses aged for more than 90 days, such as most Swiss and cheddar cheeses
- Acidophilus milk
- Buttermilk
- Cottage cheese
- Yogurt containing acidophilus
- Sherbet

You can also try these foods that have no lactose:

- Soy or rice-based drinks
- Soy products, such as soy yogurt and soy cheese
- Fluid or powdered reconstituted milk that is completely lactose-free. You can find these products in the dairy section of most grocery stores
- Nondairy creamers and frozen desserts
- Kosher foods marked "pareve," meaning meat- and milk-free
- Sorbet, but check the label. Some sorbets on the market today are made with swirled ice cream

It is important for someone on a low-lactose or lactose-free diet to find other sources of calcium. If you are on such a diet, include increased amounts of the following nondairy calcium-rich foods in your diet:

- Canned sardines and salmon with bones
- Arugula
- Calcium-fortified soy products
- Spinach
- Turnip greens
- Broccoli
- Kale

Fighting Fatigue

Fatigue is often one of the first symptoms associated with HIV disease. The disease itself, poor nutrition, opportunistic infections, fever, stress, and lack of sleep may all contribute to a loss of energy. Feeling tired and run down can worsen your emotional state, interfere with your ability to think clearly, and can make food preparation and eating a challenge. What follows are a list of ideas and a meal plan (page 58) to help make living with fatigue a little easier.

The following tips can help you fight fatigue:

- Eat breakfast every day. Start your day with a protein and complex carbohydrate to help boost energy. Try cold or hot cereal with milk, muffins with peanut butter, a bagel with cheese, yogurt with granola, leftover pizza, spaghetti, or tortillas with beans.

- Eat small meals consisting of a lean protein and complex carbohydrates frequently throughout the day. Eat every two to three hours without skipping meals. Good meal choices include turkey and mashed potatoes, stir-fried tofu with rice, three-bean salad, spaghetti, lentil burgers, tortillas and beans, and yogurt and graham crackers.

- Eat more complex carbohydrates—which help sustain energy—throughout the day. Examples include beans, tortillas, oatmeal, rice, hot and cold cereals, couscous, barley, grits, whole grain breads, breadsticks, bagels, polenta, kasha, noodles, potatoes, and pasta.

- Avoid large doses of simple sugars. These are fake energy boosters that produce a quick rush, but can ultimately increase fatigue. For example, limit doughnuts, presweetened cereals, candies, cakes, jams, jellies, syrups, and sodas.

- Drink plenty of fluids every day, especially if you're experiencing fever, diarrhea, or vomiting. Dehydration can mimic fatigue.

- Keep easy-to-prepare, simple foods on hand, such as crackers and precut cheese, eggs, frozen fruit and vegetables, breads, yogurt, cereals, peanut butter, noodles, premade frozen sauces, lean luncheon meats, and canned soups to use as sauces on fish, meat, or poultry.

- Prepare and freeze meals when your energy level is up. Freeze and store foods in single-serving containers so it's easier for you to just heat up a meal when you're tired. For salads, prepare, wash, and dry lettuce and vegetables in advance, and store in bags in the refrigerator for use throughout the week.

- Place a stool in the kitchen to sit on while preparing meals.

- Use paper plates and disposable dishes to avoid cleaning up.

- Consult your health care professional about an exercise program that's right for you. Even light exercise or slow walks may help improve energy. Don't over-exert yourself!

- Make sure you allow time in your day to simply relax or take a nap. Try taking several short naps or rests instead of one long nap.

- Keep a daily diary, noting the times of day you experience the most energy. This will help you plan your daily activities to coincide with your highest levels of energy.

- Ask for help when you need it. Take advantage of volunteer groups in your area that can provide assistance with cooking and cleanup, or will deliver meals to your home.

Alleviating Nausea and Vomiting

There are many factors that may contribute to nausea and vomiting, including headache, medication, hunger, fever, opportunistic infection, stress, overexertion, and dehydration. Learning the cause of these symptoms may help determine the best method for alleviating them.

If you are experiencing nausea and vomiting, speak with your health care professional about possible side effects from the medications you're currently taking. You may be advised to change your medication or the time you take medications to avoid side effects that interfere with your meals. Ask about antinausea medications.

Adjusting your diet also may help alleviate symptoms and, just as important, will allow you to maintain your nutritional intake. What follows are a list of ideas and a meal plan (page 60) to help make living with these symptoms a little easier.

The following tips can help you alleviate nausea and vomiting:

- Eat small meals rich in complex carbohydrates frequently throughout the day—every two to three hours.

- Eat complex carbohydrates that are plain, dry, salty, and light, such as toast; bagels; pretzels; English muffins; pita bread; rye, corn, or multigrain bread or breadsticks; plain noodles or rice; corn tortillas; and crackers. As you become less nauseated, introduce light proteins, such as baked or broiled (not fried) chicken or fish.

- Try cold entrées—such as skinless chicken, cottage cheese with fruit, or cold sandwiches—that don't have a strong aroma.

- Try bland, soft, and plain foods, such as oatmeal, white rice, baked potato or baked, skinless chicken.

- Try foods with ginger. Flat ginger ale or gingersnaps seem to help relieve nausea for many individuals. If fresh ginger is too strong, try capsules of the powdered root.

- Don't skip meals! An empty stomach may make you feel worse.

- Don't eat your favorite foods when you're nauseated. Eating these foods at this time may cause you to associate them with nausea in the future.

- Avoid fatty, greasy, or fried foods because they sit in your stomach longer. Avoid bacon, sausage, fried hamburgers, fried chicken, potato chips, French fries, and hot dogs. Limit amounts of margarine, butter, cream sauces, sour cream, cream cheese, and oil.

- Avoid very sweet foods, such as doughnuts and cakes, and very spicy foods, such as chili and other foods made with red pepper.

- Try sucking on citrus fruit wedges or citrus candies between meals, or right before you eat.

- Eat and drink foods and liquids slowly. Sip liquids—don't slurp.

- Sip liquids frequently between meals. Don't drink liquids with food because this may cause you to feel more bloated or full, which can aggravate nausea.

- Try carbonated drinks (club soda or cola) that have gone flat. Avoid fully carbonated drinks.

- Try drinks at room temperature. Avoid cold liquids that may shock your stomach.

- Keep the room in which you cook well ventilated so that cooking smells do not contribute to your nausea.

- Let someone else cook for you if the smells contribute to your nausea. Arrange to be out of the room or building when food is being cooked or prepared.

- Eat in a relaxed atmosphere and wear loose clothing.

- Rest after meals, but don't lie down for at least two hours after eating. If you need to recline, keep your head elevated at least four inches above the level of your feet.

- Try one to two tablespoons of cola syrup to settle your stomach. It's not known why this works, but it does for many people.

- Replace the electrolytes lost through vomiting. If your urine is deep yellow, this may indicate you're not taking in enough fluids. Sip electrolyte drinks (see page 38) and juices.

- Once you've stopped vomiting, reintroduce food and drink gradually. You may want to begin your nutrient intake with frozen juice cubes made in ice cube trays.

- Avoid stomach soothers such as Pepto-Bismol, Mylanta, and Maalox, unless prescribed by your health care professional. These are not specifically designed to stop nausea or vomiting caused by infections, but are instead meant to soothe a stomach irritated by excess acid. Ask your health care professional about antinausea medications that may be appropriate for you.

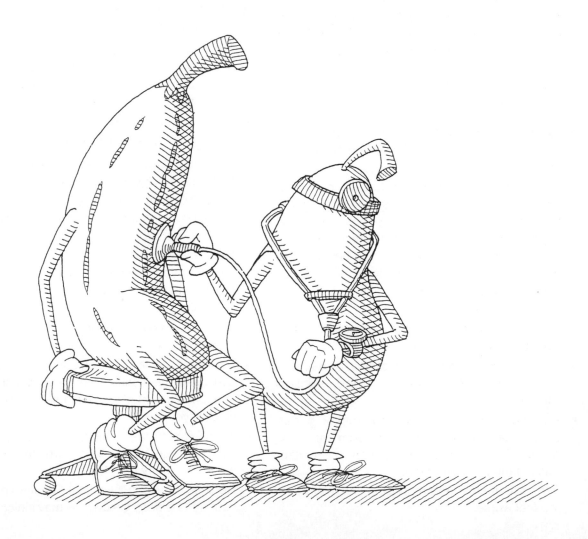

GAINING AN EDGE:
BUILDING LEAN BODY MASS

Eat, eat, eat! Now, more than ever, your body needs to maintain a weight that will help your immune system function properly. Don't wait until you experience severe weight loss before you address the problem. For a person with HIV, weight loss can occur rapidly and have serious repercussions. Moreover, it is much more difficult to gain the weight back than it is to maintain a healthy weight. Therefore, seek the advice of a health care professional as soon as you begin to experience weight loss.

You will need to alter your strategy for weight gain depending on what is causing your weight loss. You can be losing weight for a number of reasons, including increased calorie requirements due to the presence of the virus itself, your body's inability to absorb food, and loss of appetite. If you are experiencing a specific symptom that may be contributing to your weight loss, consult the pages in this section devoted to that symptom.

You should maintain a weight that is 5 to 10 percent more than your usual weight, which means you will have to eat extra calories every day. Individuals with HIV tend to lose muscle and other protein stores before losing fat stores. Therefore, try to add weight in the form of lean body mass—which consists mostly of muscle—by eating a diet with adequate amounts of protein and complex carbohydrates, and by exercising regularly. Increasing or maintaining healthy weight and lean body mass levels may help prevent opportunistic infections, provide more energy, increase toleration for medication side effects, and lessen the severity and duration of symptoms.

What follows are a list of ideas and a meal plan (page 62) to help avoid weight loss. There's also a table of food substitutions that can help provide additional calories and protein.

The following tips can help you add pounds and build lean body mass:

- Eat small meals every two to three hours throughout the day. You may find it's easier to eat small high-calorie and high-protein meals more frequently throughout the day than to try to consume one or two large meals.

- Plan menus that focus on complex carbohydrates and proteins, and try to include these choices at each meal and for each snack.

- Eat complex carbohydrates that are low in fat and high in energy. Try rice, kasha, polenta, grits, potatoes, hot and cold cereals, grains, pasta, corn, tortillas, breadsticks, and bread.

- Eat proteins, including lean meats, skinless chicken, fish, tofu, peas, and beans.

- Sip high-calorie fluids with and between meals. Instead of water, soda, or iced tea, try homemade blender drinks (see page 109), fortified milk (see page 115), fruit juices or nectars, fruit smoothies, and milk shakes.

- Keep high-calorie, low-fat snacks on hand, and try to eat a substantial snack in the evening or at bedtime. Even if you don't feel hungry, think of food as the weight-gain medicine your body needs. Remember to keep a supply of snacks with you to consume throughout the day. Good choices include dried fruits, bagels with cheese, pretzels, graham crackers, gingersnaps, muffins, and fig bars.

- Choose desserts that are low in fat but high in calories and other nutrients. Good choices include oatmeal raisin cookies, fig bars, rice pudding, stewed fruit compotes, pumpkin pie, carrot cake without frosting, muffins, breads such as applesauce or corn bread, and graham crackers.

- Choose starchy vegetables for more calories. Good choices include peas, lima beans, corn, winter squash, and potatoes.

- Never eat fruits and vegetables plain. Always add high-calorie ingredients, such as melted cheese, yogurt, or cottage cheese (see Table 5).

- Choose juices that are dark and thick, because these are generally higher in calories. When making juice from concentrate, add less water than called for in the instructions. High-calorie choices include fruit juices such as apple, cranapple, cranberry, pineapple, or grape juice, or fruit nectars such as apricot or peach nectar.

- Choose dense, whole grain, hearty breads for sandwiches and toast, and to accompany meals.

- Choose dense, whole grain cereals instead of light, presweetened ones. Good choices include granola and raisin bran.
- Take advantage of the days and times of day you feel your best by eating more at these times.
- Exercise to increase lean body mass. Do anaerobic exercises, such as lifting free weights, situps, and pushups. Never overstrain yourself. Consult your health care professional before you start an exercise program. A qualified fitness trainer can help plan an exercise program that meets your particular needs and limits.
- Keep a weight chart (see page 24). Consult your health care professional if you continue to lose weight!

Small changes in your diet can add up to big changes in your weight. For instance, instead of just eating a salad with greens, or a basic casserole or vegetable dish, add ingredients that will boost the nutrient content along with taste. Remember, it is not the best choice to add calories by simply increasing the fat in your diet. Sour cream, mayonnaise, whipped cream, ice cream, butter, and margarine all are high in calories, but are full of fat and low in nutrients. Concentrate on adding calories and protein through nutrient-dense sources rather than by adding fat. See Table 5.

Table 5. Food Addition Chart

Add	To
Milk, powdered milk, or fortified milk (substitute milk in recipes in place of water)	Hot cereals, casseroles, soups, blender drinks (page 109), puddings, custards, mashed potatoes, gravies, breads, muffins, hot cocoa
Cheese (grated, sliced, or in chunks)	Soups, sandwiches, casseroles, hamburgers, hot dogs, mashed potatoes, vegetable dishes, egg dishes, sauces, rice dishes, noodle dishes, grits, breads, muffins, burritos, couscous
Cottage cheese	Casseroles, egg dishes, quiches, soufflés, salads, noodle dishes, pancake batter, crépes, crackers, burritos, tacos, mashed potatoes
Nuts	Casseroles, egg dishes, cottage cheese, pancakes, breads, puddings, muffins, yogurt, ice cream, cookies, vegetable dishes, fruit or green salads, hot or cold cereals, trail mix, granola, peanut butter sandwiches
Fruit or dried fruit	Yogurt, hot or cold cereals, ice cream, crépes, pancakes, cottage cheese, trail mix, granola, salads, rice dishes, muffins, breads, salads, blender drinks (page 109)
Graham crackers (crumbled)	Yogurt, ice cream, hot or cold cereals, puddings, custards, fruit and dry fruit, blender drinks (page 109), peanut butter sandwiches, fruit salads

Add	To
Granola	Cookie, muffin, and bread batters; vegetables; yogurt; ice cream; puddings; custards; fruits and fruit bakes; trail mix
Hard-boiled eggs (sliced or diced)	Casseroles; pasta dishes; green, meat, or tuna salads; soups; sandwiches; rice dishes
Rice (cooked with stock instead of water)	Stir-fried dishes; burritos; tacos; casseroles; soups; stews; curries; gumbos; baked beans; scrambled eggs; stuffed bell peppers; eggplant or squash; vegetable, tuna, or egg salads; blender drinks (page 109); yogurt dishes
Wheat germ	Casseroles; meat dishes; bread, muffin, pancake, or waffle batters; fruit; hot or cold cereals; ice cream; yogurt; granola; blender drinks (page 109). Try toasted wheat germ in place of bread crumbs
Diced cooked meats or fish	Vegetable or green salads, casseroles, soups, omelets, soufflés, quiches, stuffed baked potatoes, pasta or noodle dishes
Tofu	Blender drinks (page 109), tacos, burritos, casseroles, scrambled eggs, mashed potatoes, salads, vegetables, rice dishes
Yogurt	As a topping on, or in, hot or cold cereals, pancakes, waffles, crépes, rice dishes, blender drinks (page 109)
Potatoes	Soups, salads, scrambled eggs, casseroles, bean dishes, stir-fried dishes, gumbos, curries
Legumes, such as peas and beans	Soups, casseroles, pasta dishes, burritos, tacos, stuffed baked potatoes, scrambled eggs, salads
High-calorie spreads, including jams, jellies, peanut butter, and honey	Breads, toast, sandwiches, fruits, vegetables, crackers, muffins

One-Week Meal Plan
for Chewing and Swallowing Difficulties/
Dry Mouth/Mouth and Throat Sores

2,400–2,600 calories/100–120 grams protein

Meal	Monday	Tuesday	Wednesday
Breakfast	Millet Cereal (page 78) 1 cup low-fat milk	Hot Pumpkin Cereal, modified (page 76) 1 cup applesauce 1 cup low-fat milk	1 scrambled egg 1/2 cup hash browns 1 cup fruit nectar
Snack	1 cup low-fat fruited yogurt 1/2 cup canned pears	Carrot Shake (page 114)	Apple Pie à la Mode (page 112)
Lunch	Traditional Egg Salad Sandwich, modified (page 220) 1 cup grape juice	Chicken Soup, modified (page 157) 1 cup low-fat fruited yogurt 1 cup low-fat milk	Tofu Spread, modified (page 137) 1 cup low-fat milk
Snack	1 cup low-fat cottage cheese 1/2 cup canned pears 1 cup herb tea	Deviled Eggs, modified (page 133) 1 cup herb tea	1 cup frozen low-fat yogurt 1 cup herb tea
Dinner	Potato-Zucchini Soup (page 161) 1 cup low-fat milk	Mini Meat Loaves (page 201) 1 cup mashed potato 1 cup sliced, steamed zucchini 1 cup low-fat milk	Macaroni and Cheese (page 215) 1 cup steamed mixed vegetables 1 cup low-fat milk
Snack	1 cup chocolate pudding 1 banana 1 cup herb tea	1 cup sherbet 1 cup herb tea	Creamy Berry and Chocolate Shake (page 115)

Thursday	Friday	Saturday	Sunday
1 cup cooked wheat farina 1 cup canned fruit cocktail 1 cup low-fat milk	Cottage Cheese Pancakes (page 86) 1 cup fruit nectar	Only Oatmeal (page 72) with 2 tablespoons brown sugar 1/2 cup applesauce 1 cup low-fat milk	Artichoke Eggs With Herbs (page 79) 1/2 cup applesauce 1 cup grape juice
2 slices cheese 1 cup fruit nectar	Monster Mango Mash (page 119)	Baked Rice Pudding, modified (page 234) 1 cup herb tea	1 cup low-fat cottage cheese 1 cup canned fruit cocktail 1 cup apple juice
1 cup low-fat cottage cheese 1 cup canned peaches 1 cup low-fat milk	2 cups cream of mushroom soup 1 cup apple juice	Microwave Easy Crab Delight, modified (page 199) 1 cup fruit juice	Instant Mashed Potato Soup (page 158) 1 cup low-fat milk
Banana Oat Shake (page 112)	1 cup low-fat yogurt with mashed banana and cinnamon	1 cup low-fat fruited yogurt 1 cup herb tea	Southern Buttermilk Cooler (page 123)
Turkey and Rice Casserole (page 192) 1 cup apple juice	Salmon Loaf, modified (page 196) 1 cup plain noodles 1 cup mashed cooked carrots 1 cup low-fat milk	Beef Stroganoff (page 200) 1 cup steamed mixed vegetables 1 cup low-fat milk	Broccoli Rice Bake, modified (page 177) Low-Fat Hummus (page 134) 1 cup low-fat milk
Banana Sweet Potato Pudding (page 231) 1 cup apple juice	Colonial Apple Custard (page 231) 1 cup herb tea	Honey Graham Shake (page 117)	1 cup low-fat frozen yogurt 1 cup herb tea

One-Week Meal Plan
for Alterations in Taste
2,400–2,600 calories/100–120 grams protein

Meal	Monday	Tuesday	Wednesday
Breakfast	2 slices toast with 2 teaspoons butter and 1 tablespoon orange marmalade 1 cup low-fat milk	Mexican Scrambled Eggs (page 81) 1 cup fruit juice	1 bagel with 2 tablespoons low-fat cream cheese 1 cup fruit juice
Snack	Lemon Blend (page 118)	Ginger Punch (page 116)	Cranberry Punch (page 114)
Lunch	Artichoke and Tuna Salad (page 142) 12 saltine crackers 1 cup fruit juice	1 roast beef sandwich 1 cup fruit juice	Black Bean Chili (page 163) 1 cup fruit juice
Snack	1 cup cut-up peaches 1 cup herb tea	1 cup low-fat fruited yogurt 1 cup cut-up fruit 1 cup herb tea	1 cup cut-up fruit 1 cup herb tea
Dinner	Hometown Burgers (page 201) 1 orange 1 cup low-fat milk	Greek Pasta (page 216) 1 cup fruit juice	Chicken Tandoori (page 188) 1 cup cooked couscous 1 cup steamed mixed vegetables 1 cup low-fat milk
Snack	1 cup low-fat lemon yogurt 1/4 cup granola 1 cup fruit juice	1 cup applesauce with cinnamon 1 cup milk	1 cup fruit sherbet

Thursday	Friday	Saturday	Sunday
Only Oatmeal (page 72) 1/2 cup applesauce with nutmeg 1 cup low-fat milk	1 cup dry cereal 1 piece fruit 1/2 cup low-fat milk	Scrambled Eggs With Herbs (page 83) 1 cup low-fat milk	Orangy French Toast (page 89) 1 cup low-fat milk
Orange Pineapple Delight (page 122)	5 graham crackers 1 cup apricot nectar	1 cup low-fat fruited yogurt 1 cup herb tea	5 gingersnaps 1 cup fruit juice
Low-Fat Hummus (page 134) in pita bread Fruit and Honey Spinach Salad (page 146) 1 cup low-fat milk	Mediterranean Potato (page 132) 1 orange 1 cup low-fat milk	Easy Oven Barbeque (page 184) 1 baked potato 1 cup fruit juice	1 grilled cheese sandwich 1 cup tomato soup 1 cup herb tea
1/2 cup cut-up melon 1 cup low-fat lemon yogurt 1 cup herb tea	1 cup low-fat lemon yogurt 1 banana 1 cup herb tea	1 cup pretzels 1 piece fruit 1 cup herb tea	1 piece fruit 1/2 cup low-fat cottage cheese 1 cup herb tea
Sweet and Spicy Pork Chops (page 205) 1 baked sweet potato 1 cup fruit juice	Pineapple Salmon Steaks (page 195) 1 cup cooked barley 1 cup low-fat milk	Nutty Noodles (page 218) 1 cup steamed mixed vegetables 1 cup fruit juice	Hawaiian Chicken (page 186) 1 baked potato 1 cup steamed mixed vegetables 1 cup fruit juice
5 gingersnaps 1/2 cup raisins 1 cup low-fat milk	Spicy Squash Smoothie (page 122)	Strawberry Delight (page 123)	Lemon Cake (page 228) 1 cup low-fat milk

One-Week Meal Plan
for Loss of Appetite
2,400–2,600 calories/100–120 grams protein

Note: In this meal plan, all fluids—except for milk used with dry cereal—should be drunk *between* meals.

Meal	Monday	Tuesday	Wednesday

Breakfast	1 cup dry cereal
	1 banana
	1 cup low-fat milk
		Only Oatmeal (page 72)
		1/2 cup cut-up peaches
		1 cup low-fat milk
			1 toasted bagel with
			  1 tablespoon peanut
			  butter and 2 teaspoons
			  jelly
			1 cup low-fat milk

Snack	Apricot Fruit Bars
	  (page 236)
	1 cup fruit juice
		1/2 peanut butter
		  sandwich
		1/4 cup raisins
		1 cup low-fat milk
			2 fig bars
			1 cup fruit juice

Lunch	1 roast beef sandwich
	1 cup fruit juice
		1 baked potato
		1/2 cup low-fat cottage
		  cheese
		1 cup fruit juice
			Mediterranean Potato
			  (page 132)
			1 cup fruit juice

Snack	Ginger Punch (page 116)	2 Chocolate Dreams
		  (page 233)
		1 cup low-fat milk
			1 cup low-fat fruited
			  yogurt

Dinner	1 baked skinless chicken
	  breast
	Dede's Smashed Sweet
	  Potatoes (page 174)
	1 cup low-fat milk
		Mini Meat Loaves
		  (page 201)
		Baked Barley (page 169)
		1/2 cup steamed mixed
		  vegetables
		1 cup low-fat milk
			Chicken and Artichoke
			  Casserole (page 187)
			2 slices whole wheat
			  bread
			1 cup fruit juice

Snack	5 graham crackers
	1 piece fruit
		Go Ape Shake
		  (page 117)
			Baked Rice Pudding
			  (page 234)
			1 cup fruit juice

Thursday	Friday	Saturday	Sunday
1 cup cooked kasha 1/4 cup raisins 1 cup low-fat milk	2 Lemon Yogurt Muffins (page 104) 1/2 cup low-fat cottage cheese 1 cup low-fat milk	1 cup dry cereal 1 piece fruit 1 cup low-fat milk	Crunchy Apple Granola (page 73) 1 cup low-fat milk
1 cup pretzels 1 cup fruit juice	1 banana 1 cup chocolate low-fat milk	Honey Graham Shake (page 117)	1 toasted bagel with 2 tablespoons low-fat cream cheese 1 cup low-fat milk
10 saltine crackers 1 cup tomato soup 1 slice cheese 1 cup fruit juice	Chilled Rice Salad (page 144) 2 slices bread 1 cup fruit juice	1 turkey sandwich with cheese 1 piece fruit 1 cup low-fat milk	1 cup low-fat cottage cheese 1/2 cup cut-up peaches 1 cup fruit juice
Fruit Salad Shake (page 116)	3 stalks of celery with 3 tablespoons of peanut butter 1 cup low-fat milk	Crispy Potato Snacks (page 130) 1 cup fruit juice	Cantaloupe Shake (page 113)
Bean and Cheese Enchiladas (page 210) Spanish Rice (page 172) 1 cup fruit juice	Mediterranean Baked Shrimp (page 198) 1 cup cut-up fruit 1 cup low-fat milk	McMillan's Minestrone (page 160) 5 plain crackers 1 cup low-fat milk	1 broiled pork chop 1 baked sweet potato 1 cup fruit juice
5 fig bars 1 cup low-fat milk	1 cup plain low-fat yogurt mixed with 1/4 cup dried fruit 1 cup fruit juice	1 cup low-fat frozen yogurt topped with 1/2 cup fruit 1 cup fruit juice	Easy Apple Cake (page 226) 1 cup low-fat milk

One-Week Meal Plan
for Constipation

2,400–2,600 calories/100–120 grams protein

Meal	Monday	Tuesday	Wednesday
Breakfast	1 cup bran cereal 1 banana 1 cup low-fat milk	Inside Out Vegetable Omelet (page 80) 1 cup fruit juice	Only Oatmeal (page 72) 1/4 cup raisins 1 apple 1 cup low-fat milk
Snack	1 apple 2 slices cheese 1 cup herb tea	2 Microwave Bran Muffins (page 102) 1 cup low-fat milk	Mid-Morning Pickup (page 118)
Lunch	Hearty Barley Soup (page 158) 2 slices whole wheat bread 1 cup fruit juice	1 peanut butter and banana sandwich on whole grain bread 1 cup low-fat milk	2 scrambled eggs 2 slices hearty wheat bread 1/2 cup cut-up fruit 1 cup fruit juice
Snack	1/2 cup dried fruit 1 cup herb tea	1 cup cut-up strawberries 1 cup herb tea	1 cup low-fat fruited yogurt with 2 tablespoons oat bran 2 slices whole grain toast with 1 tablespoon seeded fruit spread 1 cup herb tea
Dinner	Tamale Pie (page 203) 1 cup low-fat milk	India Casserole (page 221) 1 cup fruit juice	3 ounces skinless chicken, baked 1/2 cup cooked brown rice 1/2 cup steamed mixed vegetables 1 cup low-fat milk
Snack	Raspberry Rice Smoothie (page 121)	3 fig bars 1 cup low-fat milk	Poppy Seed Fruit Salad (page 151) 1 cup herb tea

Thursday	Friday	Saturday	Sunday
1 toasted whole wheat bagel with 1 tablespoon seeded fruit spread (such as raspberry) 1 cup low-fat milk	2 scrambled eggs 2 slices whole wheat toast with 1 tablespoon fruit spread 1 cup fruit juice	1 cup whole grain cold cereal 1/4 cup raisins 1 cup low-fat milk	1 cup whole grain hot cereal 2 cups strawberries 1 cup low-fat milk
Spinach Squares (page 136) 1 cup fruit juice	2 Prune Muffins (page 105) 1 cup low-fat milk	Vegetable Garden Dip (page 137) with 1 cup raw, cut-up vegetables 1 cup herb tea	1/4 cup mixed nuts 1 cup herb tea
Parmesan Pasta Salad, modified (page 149) 1/2 cup cut-up fruit 1 cup fruit juice	Couscous Shrimp Salad, modified (page 145) 1 cup fruit juice	1 cheese sandwich with lettuce, tomato, and cucumbers on whole wheat bread 1 cup fruit juice	Vegetarian Taco Salad (page 152) 1 cup low-fat milk
2 corn tortillas 1/2 cup whole black beans 1/4 cup cheddar cheese 1 cup herb tea	1 orange 10 wheat crackers 1 cup herb tea	Trail Mix (page 136) 1 cup herb tea	Banana Oat Shake (page 112)
Black-Eyed Pea Soup (page 156) 1 piece corn bread 1 cup fruit juice	Cornmeal Fish Fillets, modified (page 193) 2 slices whole wheat bread 1 cup steamed mixed vegetables 1 cup fruit juice	Hamburger Noodle Feast (page 202) 1 cup low-fat milk	Turkey and Rice Casserole (page 192) 1 whole grain bun sliced tomato 1 cup fruit juice
1 pear 5 graham crackers 1 cup low-fat milk	Yogurt Plus, modified (page 138) 1 cup herb tea	1 piece fruit 5 fig bars 1 cup low-fat milk	10 whole grain crackers 2 tablespoons peanut butter 1 cup fruit juice

One-Week Meal Plan for Diarrhea

2,400–2,600 calories/100–120 grams protein

Note: In this meal plan, all fluids—except for milk used with dry cereal—should be drunk *between* meals. Also, juices should be diluted, 1 part juice to 1 part water.

Meal	Monday	Tuesday	Wednesday
Breakfast	1 cup oat cereal 1 banana 1/2 cup light soymilk	Only Oatmeal (page 72) with 2 tablespoons of brown sugar 1/2 cup applesauce 2 cups diluted fruit juice	1 toasted bagel with 1 teaspoon margarine and 1 tablespoon jelly 1/2 cup canned fruit 1 hard-boiled egg 1 cup herb tea
Snack	1 bagel with 1 tablespoon jelly 2 cups diluted cranberry juice	2 slices toast with 1 teaspoon margarine 1 banana 1 cup light soymilk	Cranberry Punch (page 114) 5 graham crackers
Lunch	1 ham sandwich with 3 ounces of lean ham on white bread with mustard only 1 cup pretzels 2 cups diluted fruit juice	Tofu Egg Salad Sandwich (page 219) 2 cups chicken noodle soup 1 cup herb tea	1 baked potato, without the skin, with 1 teaspoon margarine 3 ounces turkey slices 1 cup cooked squash 2 cups diluted fruit juice
Snack	5 graham crackers Spicy Squash Smoothie, modified (page 122)	1 cup cut-up melon 3 ounces sliced turkey 1/2 cup light soymilk	2 Lemon Yogurt Muffins, modified (page 104) 1 cup light soymilk
Dinner	Sweet Potato Soup, modified (page 162) 12 saltine crackers 1 cup steamed green beans 2 cups diluted fruit juice	Sloppy Joes, modified (page 204) 1 cup steamed mixed vegetables 1 cup light soymilk	Oven Meatballs (page 203) 1 cup steamed carrots Dede's Smashed Sweet Potatoes, modified (page 174) 1 cup light soymilk
Snack	Fruited Tofu (page 131) 1/2 cup light soymilk	Baked Rice Pudding, modified (page 234) 1 cup herb tea	1 cup canned fruit 15 vanilla wafers 1 cup herb tea

Thursday	Friday	Saturday	Sunday
Banana English Muffin (page 102) 1 cup light soymilk	1 cup dry cereal 1 banana 1/2 cup light soymilk	Lactose-Free Peach Pancakes (page 87) 2 cups diluted fruit juice	Scrambled Tofu, modified (page 84) 2 slices toast with 1 teaspoon margarine and 1 tablespoon jam 2 cups diluted fruit juice
Spicy Squash Smoothie, modified (page 122)	15 vanilla wafers 1 pear, skin removed 1 hard-boiled egg 1 cup herb tea	15 saltines 3 slices of ham 1 cup herb tea	Strawberry Delight, modified (page 123)
1 turkey sandwich on white bread with mustard only 1 cup canned fruit 2 cups diluted fruit juice	1 cup cooked noodles 1/2 cup marinara sauce 3 slices French bread with 1 teaspoon margarine 1 cup light soymilk	Low-Fat Hummus (page 134) in pita bread 1 banana 2 cups diluted fruit juice	2 cups chicken noodle soup 15 plain crackers 2 cups diluted fruit juice 1 cup cut-up melon
15 plain crackers 1 cup cut-up melon 1 cup light soymilk	Honey Graham Shake, modified (page 117)	1 cup cooked wheat farina with 1 tablespoon brown sugar 1 cup applesauce 1 cup herb tea	5 graham crackers 1 cup applesauce 1 cup light soymilk
Easy Chicken Teriyaki (page 185) 1 cup cooked couscous 1 cup steamed green beans 1 cup light soymilk	Oven Fried Scallops (page 197) 1 cup cooked white rice 1 cup steamed mixed vegetables 2 cups diluted fruit juice	Tofu Rice Burgers, modified (page 222) 1 cup cut-up melon 1 cup light soymilk	Lemon-Soy Chicken (page 188) 1 cup sliced, steamed zucchini 1 baked potato, without skin, with 1 teaspoon margarine 1 cup light soymilk
1 cup pretzels 1 cup cut-up strawberries and bananas 2 cups diluted fruit juice	Blueberry Crisp, modified (page 237) 1 cup light soymilk	Pear Icey (page 121)	Custard Bread Pudding, modified (page 232) 1 cup light soymilk

One-Week Meal Plan
for Fatigue

2,400–2,600 calories/100–120 grams protein

Meal	Monday	Tuesday	Wednesday
Breakfast	2 packages instant hot cereal 1 cup low-fat milk	Quick Cinnamon Spread on toast (page 135) 1 piece fruit 1 cup low-fat milk	1 cup dry cereal 1 piece fruit 1 cup low-fat milk
Snack	1 banana with 2 tablespoons peanut butter 1 cup low-fat milk	1 piece fruit 1/2 cup low-fat cottage cheese 1 cup herb tea	Banana Oat Shake (page 112)
Lunch	Cheesy Pasta Primavera (page 215) 1 cup fruit juice	Double Nut Sandwich (page 216) 1 cup low-fat milk	1 cup low-fat cottage cheese 1/2 cup cut-up melon 10 plain crackers 1 cup fruit juice
Snack	15 plain crackers 2 slices cheese 1 cup herb tea	1 baked potato with 2 tablespoons low-fat plain yogurt 1 cup fruit juice	5 fig bars 1 cup low-fat yogurt 1 cup herb tea
Dinner	Turkey and Rice Casserole (page 192) 1 cup steamed corn kernels 1 cup fruit juice	Sloppy Joes (see page 204) 1 cup steamed peas 1 cup low-fat milk	Cottage Cheese Potato (page 130) 1 cup steamed mixed vegetables 1 cup low-fat milk
Snack	1 Chocolate Dream (page 233) 1 cup low-fat milk	1 cup sherbet 1 cup herb tea	1/2 turkey sandwich on whole grain bread 1 cup fruit juice

Thursday	Friday	Saturday	Sunday
Breakfast Rice (page 75) 1 cup fruit juice	Breakfast Sandwich (page 82) 1 cup low-fat milk	Baked Egg Sandwich (page 78) 1 cup fruit juice	1 cup low-fat fruited yogurt with 1 tablespoon wheat germ 1 banana 1 cup fruit juice
1 cup low-fat fruited yogurt 1 cup herb tea	Strawberry Delight (page 123)	1 cup canned fruit 1/2 cup low-fat cottage cheese 1 cup herb tea	1 toasted bagel with 2 tablespoons peanut butter 1 cup low-fat milk
1 ham sandwich 1 piece fruit 1 cup low-fat milk	Crunchy English Muffins (page 129) 1 cup fruit juice	1 cheese sandwich 1 cup fruit juice	Corn and Pea Salad (page 141) 1 cup, herb tea
2 Microwave Bran Muffins (page 102) 1 cup low-fat milk	Four-Bean Salad (page 143) 1 cup fruit juice	5 graham crackers 1 cup herb tea	1/4 cup dried fruit 2 tablespoons nuts 1 cup herb tea
Cheesy Bean and Rice Casserole (page 212) 2 flour tortillas 1 cup fruit juice	Tuna Bake (page 196) 1 cup steamed corn kernels 1 cup low-fat milk	Mexican Baked Chicken With Beans (page 189) 1 cup steamed green beans 1 cup fruit juice	Italian Bulgur Bake (page 214) 1 cup steamed mixed vegetables 1 cup low-fat milk
Microwave Fruit Pudding (page 234) 1 cup herb tea	1 banana 1 cup low-fat milk	Easy Apple Cake (page 226) 1 cup low-fat milk	2 Banana Grahams (page 128) 1 cup fruit juice

One-Week Meal Plan for Nausea and Vomiting

2,400–2,600 calories/100–120 grams protein

Note: In this meal plan, all fluids—except for milk used with dry cereal—should be drunk *between* meals.

Meal	Monday	Tuesday	Wednesday
Breakfast	Only Oatmeal (page 72) with 2 tablespoons brown sugar and 2 tablespoons raisins 1 cup low-fat milk	1 cup dry cereal 1 banana 1 cup low-fat milk	1 Pumpkin Raisin Muffin (page 106) 1 cup low-fat lemon yogurt 1 cup low-fat milk
Snack	1/2 cup low-fat cottage cheese 1/2 cup cut-up melon 1 cup herb tea	Lemon Blend (page 118) 5 gingersnaps	1 toasted English muffin with 1 tablespoon apricot preserves 1/2 cup low-fat cottage cheese 1 cup herb tea
Lunch	1 roast beef sandwich 1/2 cup pretzels 1 cup low-fat milk	1 ham sandwich 1/2 cup pretzels 1 cup fruit juice	Low-Fat Hummus (page 134) in pita bread 1 cup low-fat milk
Snack	Cereal Party Mix (page 128) 1 cup fruit juice	1 cup chicken noodle soup 10 plain crackers 1 orange 1 cup herb tea	Monster Mango Mash (page 119)
Dinner	Easy Tomato and Rice Soup (page 157) 2 pieces of French bread 1 cup low-fat milk	Chicken à la Orange (page 184) 1 baked sweet potato 1/2 cup steamed peas 1 cup low-fat milk	Pork Chop Baked With Apples and Sweet Potatoes (page 205) 1 cup fruit juice
Snack	Peach Smoothie (page 120)	Lemon Gingerbread Cake (page 229) 1 cup fruit juice	1 cup low-fat fruited yogurt 5 graham crackers 1 cup herb tea

Thursday	Friday	Saturday	Sunday
1 cup cooked grits 1/2 cup canned peaches, packed in either juice or water 1 cup low-fat milk	1 cup dry cereal 1/2 cup cut-up fruit 1 cup low-fat milk	Oatmeal Pancakes (page 88) 1 cup applesauce 1 cup low-fat milk	Hot Pumpkin Cereal (page 76) 1 cup low-fat milk
Ginger Punch (page 116)	2 pieces of toast with 1 tablespoon apricot preserves 1 cup low-fat milk	1 piece fruit 1 cup pretzels 1 cup fruit juice	2 pieces of toast with 1 tablespoon orange marmalade 1 cup low-fat yogurt 1 cup herb tea
1 turkey sandwich 1 cup fruit juice	Tofu Egg Salad Sandwich (page 219) 1/2 cup pretzels 1 cup fruit juice	1 baked potato 1/2 cup low-fat cottage cheese 1 cup cut-up, steamed broccoli 1 cup fruit juice	Potato-Zucchini Soup (page 161) 10 plain crackers 1 cup fruit juice
Banana English Muffin (page 102) 1 cup fruit juice	Carrot Shake (page 114) 5 gingersnaps	Tropical Fruit Salad (page 148) 1 cup low-fat milk	Blueberry Orange Whip (page 113)
Lemon-Soy Chicken (page 188) 1 cup cooked brown rice 1 cup fruit juice	Poached Fish (page 194) 1 baked potato 1 cup steamed mixed vegetables 1 cup fruit juice	Oven Meatballs (page 203) 1 cup cooked brown rice 1/2 cup steamed mixed vegetables 1 cup low-fat milk	Tofu Rice Burgers, modified (page 222) 1 cup steamed corn kernels 1 cup fruit juice
1 cup low-fat cottage cheese 1 cup cut-up fruit 5 graham crackers 1 cup herb tea	Lemon Cake, modified (page 228) 1 cup low-fat milk	5 fig bars 1 cup herb tea	1 cup pretzels 1 banana 1/2 cup low-fat cottage cheese 1 cup herb tea

One-Week Meal Plan
for Weight Gain

3,000–3,500 calories/125–145 grams protein

Meal	Monday	Tuesday	Wednesday
Breakfast	Only Oatmeal (page 72) with 2 tablespoons raisins and 1 tablespoon brown sugar 1 cup low-fat milk	2 cups whole grain dry cereal 1 cup low-fat milk 1 piece fruit	Crunchy Apple Granola (page 73) 1 banana 1 cup low-fat milk
Snack	1 banana 1 cup fruit nectar	1 cup low-fat fruited yogurt 6 graham crackers 1 cup herb tea	5 fig bars 1 orange 1 cup low-fat milk
Lunch	Toasty Chicken Salad Sandwiches (page 190) 1 piece fruit 1 cup low-fat milk	1 peanut butter and raisin sandwich 1 cup cut-up strawberries 1 cup low-fat milk	1 roast beef sandwich 1 cup fruit juice
Snack	Apple Pie à la Mode (page 112)	2 Cheesecake Sandwiches (page 129) 1 cup fruit juice	Banana Oat Shake (page 112)
Dinner	India Casserole (page 221) 1 cup fruit juice	Mexican Baked Chicken With Beans (page 189) 2 flour tortillas 1/2 avocado, sliced 1 cup fruit juice	Turkey Burger (page 191) Crispy Potato Snacks (page 130) 1 cup steamed mixed vegetables 1 cup low-fat milk
Snack	1 toasted bagel 2 slices cheese 1 cup low-fat fruited yogurt 1 cup herb tea	Creamy Berry and Chocolate Shake (page 115)	1 cheese sandwich 1 cup fruit juice

Thursday	Friday	Saturday	Sunday
Breakfast Rice (page 75) 1 cup fruit juice	1 cup low-fat cottage cheese 1/2 cup pineapple chunks 1 toasted bagel with 1 tablespoon jam 1 cup low-fat milk	Buckwheat Pancakes (page 85) with 1/2 cup warmed applesauce and cinnamon 1 banana 1 cup low-fat milk	Orangy French Toast (page 89) 2 tablespoons maple syrup 1 cup fruit juice
2 slices toast with 2 tablespoons peanut butter and 1 tablespoon jam 1 cup low-fat milk	1 cup pretzels 1 cup fruit juice	Nutty Whip (page 119)	2 slices cheese 12 plain crackers 1 cup herb tea
1 baked potato 2 slices cheese 1 cup cut-up, steamed broccoli 1 cup fruit juice	Double Nut Sandwich (page 216) 1 cup low-fat milk	Vegetarian Taco Salad (page 152) 1 cup cut-up fruit 1 cup low-fat milk	1 tuna salad sandwich 1 cup fruit juice
Nutty Banana Pops (page 135) 1/2 cup low-fat cottage cheese 1 cup low-fat milk	Cereal Party Mix (page 128) 1 cup herb tea	1 cup low-fat fruited yogurt 1 cup cut-up fruit 1 cup herb tea	Raspberry Rice Smoothie (page 121)
Microwave Lentil Burritos (page 219) 1 cup fruit juice	Baked Parmesan Fish Fillets (page 194) 1 baked potato with 2 tablespoons sour cream 1 cup steamed mixed vegetables 1 cup low-fat milk	Hamburger Noodle Feast (page 202) 1 cup steamed mixed vegetables 1 cup low-fat milk	Panama Pasta (page 217) 2 slices French bread with 2 teaspoons butter 1 cup low-fat milk
Cantaloupe Shake (page 113)	2 Strawberry Muffins (page 107) 1 cup fruit juice	5 fig bars 1 piece fruit 1 cup low-fat milk	Zucchini Chocolate Cake (page 230) 1 cup low-fat milk

Part Two

The
Recipes

The kitchen-tested recipes in this part are both good for you and just plain good–
ask our tasters! We cover everything: wholesome breakfasts, sumptuous breads,
tasty blender beverages and snacks, delightful salads, hearty soups, wonderful side
dishes, satisfying entrées (both with meat and without), and divine desserts. If you're not
an expert chef, the accompanying table of common cooking terms may be useful.

To help you meet your nutritional goals, each recipe comes complete with a calorie
count, as well as with the amounts of carbohydrate, protein, and fat. The chart at the
beginning of each section lets you know which recipes in that section can help alleviate
the specific HIV symptoms discussed in Using Diet to Help Alleviate HIV Symptoms.
In addition, each recipe itself lists the symptoms it was designed to help soothe, and
some recipes come with modifications so that a recipe can be adapted to suit a specific
symptom.

Of course, you should feel free to adjust ingredients according to your tastes and
tolerances. When adjusting recipes, be sure to take into account any changes this may
have on that recipe's nutrition information.

Common Cooking Terms

These are cooking terms you will encounter in this book.

Bake. To cook, either covered or uncovered, in an oven.

Baste. To keep foods moist during cooking by pouring liquid, such as meat drippings, over them.

Beat. To make a mixture creamy, smooth, or filled with air by whipping it in a brisk motion. This can be done either by hand with either a wire whisk or a spoon, or by using an electric mixer.

Blend. To stir two or more ingredients together until they are smooth and uniform throughout.

Boil. To cook at a boiling temperature. Boiling occurs when bubbles form rapidly, rising continually and breaking when they reach the surface of the liquid.

Broil. To cook a food by placing it on a rack located directly under the source of heat.

Chill. To put food in the refrigerator until it is cold throughout.

Chop. To cut food in pieces about the size of small peas.

Cool. To remove a food from the source of heat and either let it stand at room temperature or place it in the refrigerator until it reaches the desired temperature.

Cream. To combine a dry ingredient such as sugar with an oily ingredient such as butter by lightly working the ingredients together with either the fingers or the back of a wooden spoon.

Dice. To cut food in small cubes that are all of the same size and shape.

Drizzle. To slowly pour a very thin stream of liquid lightly over food.

Dust. To sprinkle food very lightly with a dry ingredient, such as sugar or flour.

Fillet. To cut meat, chicken, or fish from the bone.

Flour. To coat a greased dish with flour, tapping out any excess.

Fold. To gently work an ingredient such as fruit into a batter, using either the fingers or a large spoon. The bowl should be turned as the ingredient is folded in.

Grate. To turn a solid food to fine shreds by either rubbing it against a hand grater or placing it in a food processor.

Grill. To cook food on a rack directly over the source of heat.

Marinate. To make foods more flavorful or tender by allowing them to stand in a liquid for several hours or overnight. Food should always be marinated in the refrigerator.

Mince. To chop food into very fine pieces.

Mix. To stir ingredients until they are very well blended.

Parboil. To cook a food in a boiling liquid until it is partly cooked.

Preheat. To set an oven or broiler at the desired temperature 15 to 30 minutes before use, so that the desired temperature is reached before the food is put in to cook.

Purée. To blend a food until it is smooth and uniform throughout.

Sauté. To cook food quickly in melted butter or oil until tender.

Scramble. To prepare eggs by gently stirring them with a fork.

Simmer. To cook food in liquid that is just below the boiling point.

Steam. To cook food in steam. Usually, food is put on a rack or in a perforated pan, and placed in a covered container that has a small amount of boiling liquid in the bottom.

Stir. To thoroughly combine two or more ingredients using a spoon.

Stir-fry. To quickly sauté meat or vegetables while stirring constantly in a hot wok or frying pan.

Toast. To brown by means of dry heat, either in an oven or in a toaster.

Toss. To mix lightly and gently, usually with a lifting motion.

Healthy Start Breakfasts

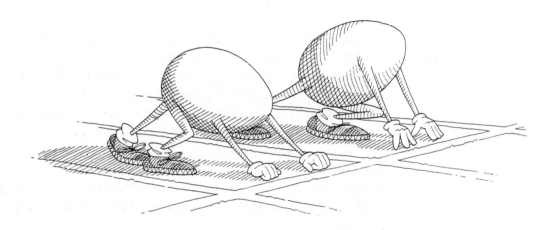

You guessed it, your mom was right. Breakfast is the most important meal of the day. Never skip breakfast! Everyone needs this morning infusion of nutrients in order to fuel the body. Breakfast should include complex carbohydrates and proteins to provide the energy and stamina needed for the coming day.

We have provided a variety of breakfast choices, including hot and cold cereals, egg dishes, pancake variations, and truly tempting French toasts. But don't feel you have to stick to the choices in this section for your breakfast. If you wake up craving pizza, by all means indulge. Just keep in mind that you want the bulk of your nutrients at this meal to provide you with lasting energy—so don't fill up on refined sugars.

You can add to the nutrients and calories at breakfast by topping cereal, pancakes, and French toast with favorite fruits or nuts, trail mix, applesauce, peanut butter, or low-fat yogurt. Egg dishes can be enlivened by adding leftover vegetables, potatoes, spices, or salsa.

Recipe-by-Symptoms Chart

Different recipes in this section are designed to address different symptoms that commonly occur in people with HIV disease. This chart can help you find recipes to ease your symptoms. You'll note that some recipes address multiple symptoms.

ALTERATIONS IN TASTE	Crunchy Apple Granola, Hot Pumpkin Cereal, Lactose-Free Peach Pancakes, Mexican Scrambled Eggs, Only Oatmeal, Orangy French Toast, Oven Omelet, Scrambled Eggs With Herbs, Scrambled Tofu
CHEWING AND SWALLOWING DIFFICULTIES	Artichoke Eggs With Herbs, Baked Oatmeal, Breakfast Rice (modified), Cottage Cheese Pancakes, Hot Pumpkin Cereal (modified), Inside Out Vegetable Omelet, Lactose-Free Peach Pancakes, Mexican Scrambled Eggs (modified), Millet Cereal, Oatmeal Pancakes, Only Oatmeal, Orangy French Toast, Oven Omelet, Scrambled Eggs With Herbs, Scrambled Tofu
CONSTIPATION	Breakfast Rice, Buckwheat Pancakes, Cottage Cheese Pancakes, Crunchy Apple Granola, Fruited Grits, Hot Pumpkin Cereal, Inside Out Vegetable Omelet, Mexican Scrambled Eggs, Millet Cereal, Only Oatmeal
DIARRHEA	Artichoke Eggs With Herbs (modified), Baked Oatmeal (modified), Fruited Grits (modified), Hot Pumpkin Cereal (modified), Inside Out Vegetable Omelet (modified), Lactose-Free Peach Pancakes, Oatmeal Pancakes (modified), Only Oatmeal, Orangy French Toast (modified), Scrambled Eggs With Herbs (modified), Scrambled Tofu (modified)
DRY MOUTH	Artichoke Eggs With Herbs, Breakfast Rice (modified), Cottage Cheese Pancakes, Fruited Grits, Hot Pumpkin Cereal, Lactose-Free Peach Pancakes, Millet Cereal, Oatmeal Pancakes, Only Oatmeal, Orangy French Toast, Oven Omelet, Scrambled Eggs With Herbs, Scrambled Tofu

FATIGUE

Baked Egg Sandwich, Baked Oatmeal, Breakfast Rice, Breakfast Sandwich, Buckwheat Pancakes, Cottage Cheese Pancakes, Crunchy Apple Granola, Fruited Grits, Inside Out Vegetable Omelet, Mexican Scrambled Eggs, Millet Cereal, Oatmeal Pancakes, Only Oatmeal, Oven Omelet, Scrambled Eggs With Herbs

LOSS OF APPETITE

Artichoke Eggs With Herbs, Baked Egg Sandwich, Baked Oatmeal, Breakfast Rice, Buckwheat Pancakes, Crunchy Apple Granola, Fruited Grits, Inside Out Vegetable Omelet, Lactose-Free Peach Pancakes, Millet Cereal, Oatmeal Pancakes, Only Oatmeal, Scrambled Tofu

MOUTH AND THROAT SORES

Artichoke Eggs With Herbs, Baked Oatmeal, Breakfast Rice (modified), Cottage Cheese Pancakes, Fruited Grits (modified), Hot Pumpkin Cereal (modified), Lactose-Free Peach Pancakes, Mexican Scrambled Eggs (modified), Millet Cereal, Oatmeal Pancakes, Only Oatmeal, Oven Omelet, Scrambled Eggs With Herbs

NAUSEA AND VOMITING

Artichoke Eggs With Herbs (modified), Buckwheat Pancakes, Fruited Grits (modified), Hot Pumpkin Cereal, Inside Out Vegetable Omelet (modified), Lactose-Free Peach Pancakes, Oatmeal Pancakes, Only Oatmeal, Orangy French Toast (modified), Scrambled Eggs With Herbs

WEIGHT GAIN

Baked Egg Sandwich, Baked Oatmeal, Breakfast Rice, Breakfast Sandwich, Buckwheat Pancakes, Cottage Cheese Pancakes, Crunchy Apple Granola, Fruited Grits, Hot Pumpkin Cereal, Inside Out Vegetable Omelet, Mexican Scrambled Eggs, Millet Cereal, Oatmeal Pancakes, Only Oatmeal, Orangy French Toast, Oven Omelet, Scrambled Eggs With Herbs, Scrambled Tofu

Only Oatmeal

Yield: 1 serving
Preparation time: 10 to 20 minutes

½ cup water

½ cup low-fat milk

1 teaspoon salt

½ cup oats, quick-cooking or rolled

Oatmeal is a high-energy food that's good anytime. To make the following recipe richer, use milk instead of milk and water. You can make as many servings at a time as you wish—just multiply the ingredients by the number of servings you desire.

1. Place the water and milk in a small saucepan, and bring to a rolling boil. Add the salt and oats, and lower the heat to medium.

2. Cook, uncovered, for 5 minutes, stirring occasionally. Remove from the heat. If you are using quick-cooking oats, the cereal is ready. If you are using rolled oats, cover the saucepan and set aside for 15 minutes. The longer the oats stand, the creamier they will be.

3. Add your favorite topping from the list below, or be creative according to your tolerances. Serve immediately.

NUTRITION INFORMATION (PER SERVING, WITHOUT TOPPING):
Calories: 215   Fat: 5 g   Carbohydrate: 32 g   Protein: 11 g

---

Good for every symptom with topping variations.

Microwave Cooking

Place all of the ingredients in a microwave-safe bowl. Cover with waxed paper, and cook on high power for 2 to 5 minutes. Serve the quick-cooking oats immediately. If using rolled oats, cover and set aside for 15 minutes before serving.

Topping Variations

Suggested toppings when experiencing alterations in taste: lemon yogurt, dried pineapple or apricots, canned or fresh chopped citrus fruits, apricot preserves, cherries, cinnamon, and nutmeg.

Suggested toppings when experiencing constipation: nuts, seeds, dried fruit, wheat germ, seeded preserves, bran, chopped fresh fruit, coconut flakes, cinnamon, and nutmeg.

Suggested toppings when experiencing diarrhea: unsweetened applesauce, puréed or canned fruit, banana, light soymilk, oat bran, brown sugar, cinnamon, and nutmeg.

Suggested toppings when experiencing fatigue or loss of appetite, or for weight gain: peanut butter, jam or jelly, nuts, seeds, yogurt, raisins, dried fruit, chopped fresh fruit, wheat germ, oat bran, coconut flakes, milk, brown sugar, cinnamon, and nutmeg.

Suggested toppings when experiencing dry mouth, chewing and swallowing difficulties, or mouth and throat sores: yogurt, creamy peanut butter, jam or jelly, puréed fruit, applesauce, banana, low-fat milk, brown sugar, maple syrup, cinnamon, and nutmeg.

Suggested toppings when experiencing nausea and vomiting: chopped fresh fruit, applesauce, puréed or canned fruits, dried fruit, plain low-fat yogurt, low-fat milk, cinnamon, and nutmeg.

Modification

If experiencing diarrhea, omit the low-fat milk and use $\frac{1}{2}$ cup light soymilk.

MODIFIED NUTRITION INFORMATION:

Calories: 200   Fat: 4 g   Carbohydrate: 35 g   Protein: 9 g

Crunchy Apple Granola

Yield: 10 servings
Preparation time: 20 minutes

1 ½ cups rolled oats

1 cup chopped walnuts

1 cup Grape Nuts cereal

1 cup chopped dried apples

½ cup brown sugar, firmly packed

This cereal is easy to make ahead of time. Serve with milk, stir into yogurt, or sprinkle on top of ice cream.

1. Preheat oven to 350°F.

2. Place all the ingredients in a large bowl, and mix thoroughly. Coat a cookie sheet with nonstick cooking spray, and spread the mixture evenly on the sheet.

3. Bake 10 minutes, or until the cereal is crunchy; stir 3 times while the cereal is cooking. Remove from the oven, and let cool. Store in an airtight container.

NUTRITION INFORMATION (PER SERVING):

Calories: 285   Fat: 10 g   Carbohydrate: 45 g   Protein: 8 g

---

Good for alterations in taste, constipation, fatigue,
loss of appetite, and weight gain.

Baked Oatmeal

Yield: 4 servings
Preparation time: 35 minutes

¼ cup unsweetened applesauce

½ cup brown sugar, firmly packed

2 eggs plus 2 egg whites

1 cup low-fat milk

2 teaspoons baking powder

1 teaspoon salt

3 cups rolled oats

No one can stop eating this dish once it's out of the oven! Top with warmed applesauce to make it even more irresistible. Leftovers make a great snack when you're on the run.

1. Preheat the oven to 350°F.

2. Place the applesauce, sugar, eggs, and milk in a small bowl, and mix thoroughly. Place the baking powder, salt, and oats in a large bowl, and mix completely. Add the applesauce mixture to the oat mixture, mixing thoroughly.

3. Coat an 8-inch square baking pan with nonstick cooking spray. Pour evenly into the pan. Bake 30 minutes, or until the top is firm to the touch.

NUTRITION INFORMATION (PER SERVING):

Calories: 420   Fat: 8 g   Carbohydrate: 73 g   Protein: 17 g

---

Good for chewing and swallowing difficulties, fatigue, loss of appetite, mouth and throat sores, and weight gain.

Modification

If experiencing diarrhea, omit the low-fat milk and use 1 cup light soymilk.

MODIFIED NUTRITION INFORMATION:

Calories: 415   Fat: 7 g   Carbohydrate: 74 g   Protein: 15 g

---

Breakfast Rice

Yield: 2 servings
Preparation time: 10 to 15 minutes

½ cup cooked brown rice

2 cups low-fat milk

½ cup raisins

⅛ teaspoon ground cinnamon

⅛ teaspoon ground nutmeg

¼ cup maple syrup, honey, or molasses

Start your day with high-energy breakfast rice. If you don't have instant rice, use leftovers or regular brown rice. If you're cooking regular rice from scratch, you will need to adjust the cooking time accordingly; see page 213 for cooking instructions.

1. Place the rice, milk, and raisins in a medium-sized saucepan, and bring to a boil.

2. Cover, reduce the heat to medium, and simmer until the rice is cooked, about 5 to 10 minutes.

3. Place the cooked rice, the spices, and the maple syrup, honey, or molasses in a medium-sized bowl, and mix thoroughly. Serve warm.

NUTRITION INFORMATION (PER SERVING):

Calories: 450   Fat: 6 g   Carbohydrate: 94 g   Protein: 12 g

---

Good for constipation, fatigue, loss of appetite, and weight gain.

Modification

If experiencing chewing and swallowing difficulties, dry mouth, or mouth and throat sores, omit the raisins and add ½ cup chopped fresh or canned fruit, as tolerated.

MODIFIED NUTRITION INFORMATION:

Calories: 460   Fat: 6 g   Carbohydrate: 96 g   Protein: 12 g

---

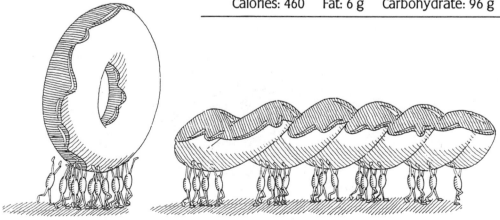

Hot Pumpkin Cereal

Yield: 2 servings
Preparation time: 20 minutes

½ cup dry wheat farina or
   rolled oats

½ cup evaporated skim milk

1 cup canned pumpkin purée

½ teaspoon ground cinnamon

½ teaspoon ground allspice

¼ tablespoon ground coriander

2 tablespoons raisins

2 tablespoons honey

This cereal reminds us of the holidays. It is very soothing, yet hearty.

1. Place all the ingredients in a medium-sized saucepan over medium heat. Cook uncovered, stirring occasionally, for about 10 minutes, or until the mixture thickens. Serve immediately.

NUTRITION INFORMATION (PER SERVING):
Calories: 225   Fat: less than 1 g   Carbohydrate: 50 g   Protein: 8 g

Good for alterations in taste, constipation, dry mouth,
nausea and vomiting, and weight gain.

Modification

If experiencing chewing and swallowing difficulties, diarrhea, or mouth and throat sores, omit the skim milk and raisins, and use ½ cup light soymilk or lactose-reduced milk and ¼ cup unsweetened applesauce. Use spices as tolerated.

MODIFIED NUTRITION INFORMATION:
Calories: 185   Fat: 1 g   Carbohydrate: 43 g   Protein: 4 g

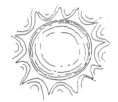

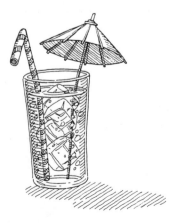

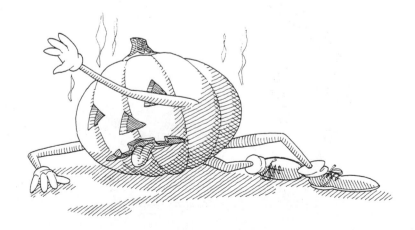

Fruited Grits

Yield: 2 servings
Preparation time: 10 minutes

1 ¼ cups low-fat milk

¾ cup instant grits

½ cup raisins

1 tablespoon sugar

½ teaspoon ground cinnamon

¼ teaspoon ground nutmeg

¼ cup chopped nuts

If raisins aren't to your liking, try any other type of dried fruit to boost the calories of this spicy-sweet hot breakfast. It's good any time of the day.

1. Place milk in a small saucepan over low heat, and heat just until bubbles form at the sides of the saucepan. Stir often to avoid scorching the milk.

2. Place the other ingredients in a small bowl, and mix thoroughly.

3. Pour the hot milk over the grits mixture. Let stand a few minutes, until the grits are softened, before serving.

NUTRITION INFORMATION (PER SERVING):

Calories: 385   Fat: 12 g   Carbohydrate: 62 g   Protein: 12 g

---

Good for constipation, dry mouth, fatigue,
loss of appetite, and weight gain.

Modification

If experiencing diarrhea, mouth and throat sores, or nausea and vomiting, omit the low-fat milk, raisins, and nuts. Use 1 ¼ cups light soymilk or lactose-reduced milk, and add 1 ripe banana, sliced.

MODIFIED NUTRITION INFORMATION:

Calories: 200   Fat: 4 g   Carbohydrate: 40 g   Protein: 7 g

Millet Cereal

Yield: 2 servings
Preparation time: 40 minutes

½ cup whole, hulled millet

1 ½ cups low-fat milk

1 teaspoon salt

¼ cup honey

Try this wonderfully different grain for a change-of-pace breakfast. For more information on millet, see page 168.

1. Place the millet, milk, and salt in a small saucepan, and bring to a boil. Cover, reduce the heat to medium, and let simmer 30 minutes, or until the millet is cooked.

2. Stir in the honey before serving. Serve warm.

NUTRITION INFORMATION (PER SERVING):

Calories: 410   Fat: 6 g   Carbohydrate: 79 g   Protein: 12 g

---

Good for chewing and swallowing difficulties, constipation, dry mouth, fatigue, loss of appetite, mouth and throat sores, and weight gain.

Baked Egg Sandwich

Yield: 1 sandwich
Preparation time: 20 minutes

1 egg

1 tablespoon low-fat milk

1 teaspoon chopped
well-washed parsley

1 teaspoon mayonnaise

2 slices whole grain bread

2 thick slices well-washed
tomato

1 slice cheddar cheese

½ teaspoon ground paprika

This sandwich can be a meal in itself, but it also makes a hearty snack. Always choose the most dense bread you can find to get the most calories, protein, and vitamins.

1. Preheat the broiler, or use a toaster oven.

2. Place the egg, milk, and parsley in a small bowl, and beat together thoroughly. Pour into an 8-inch frying pan coated with nonstick cooking spray over medium heat, and scramble until very firm.

3. Spread the mayonnaise on one slice of the bread, and top with the scrambled egg, tomato, and cheese. Sprinkle with the paprika.

4. Place both pieces of bread under the broiler or in the toaster oven until the cheese melts, about 2 minutes. Make a sandwich, and serve immediately.

NUTRITION INFORMATION (PER SANDWICH):

Calories: 360   Fat: 19 g   Carbohydrate: 29 g   Protein: 20 g

---

Good for fatigue, loss of appetite, and weight gain.

Artichoke Eggs With Herbs

Yield: 2 servings
Preparation time: 20 to 25 minutes

1 can (15 ounces) artichoke hearts in water, drained

2 tablespoons chopped pimientos

¼ teaspoon dried marjoram, or 1/2 teaspoon chopped fresh

1 tablespoon chopped well-washed parsley

1 tablespoon low-fat milk

2 eggs

½ teaspoon salt

Artichokes are a rich source of vitamin C, and this is a delicious way to use them.

1. Chop the artichoke hearts coarsely and place in a medium-sized bowl. Add the pimientos, marjoram, and parsley, and mix thoroughly. Set aside.

2. Place the milk, eggs, and salt in a separate bowl, and beat together thoroughly. Pour into an 8-inch frying pan coated with nonstick cooking spray over medium heat.

3. When eggs have started to set, add the artichoke mixture and lift up the eggs with a spatula to allow liquid to run underneath. As the bottom sets, turn the eggs over, and continue cooking until very firm. Serve immediately.

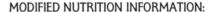

NUTRITION INFORMATION (PER SERVING):

Calories: 250   Fat: 11 g   Carbohydrate: 23 g   Protein: 19 g

Good for chewing and swallowing difficulties, dry mouth, loss of appetite, and mouth and throat sores.

Modification

If experiencing diarrhea or nausea and vomiting, omit the low-fat milk and whole eggs, and use 1 tablespoon light soymilk or lactose-reduced milk and 4 egg whites.

MODIFIED NUTRITION INFORMATION:

Calories: 165   Fat: 1 g   Carbohydrate: 22 g   Protein: 21 g

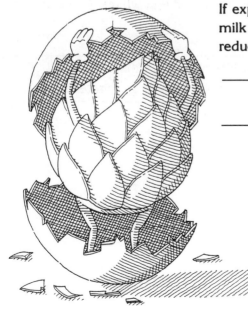

Inside Out Vegetable Omelet

Yield: 2 servings
Preparation time: 30 minutes

1 teaspoon olive oil

½ cup chopped onion

1 clove garlic, minced

1 cup chopped well-washed
    tomato

½ cup chopped well-washed
    green bell pepper

1 cup sliced well-washed
    mushrooms

4 eggs

½ teaspoon salt

½ teaspoon black pepper

½ teaspoon ground paprika

1 teaspoon dried oregano, or 1
    tablespoon chopped fresh

½ cup grated cheese of your
    choice

This is a great dish if you want to use up leftover vegetables. Use whatever ingredients suit your taste.

1. Place the oil in a large frying pan over medium heat. Add the onion and garlic, and sauté for 3 minutes. Add the tomato, green pepper, and mushrooms, and sauté for an additional 2 minutes.

2. Break the eggs into the frying pan over the vegetables, and sprinkle with the spices and cheese. Cook over medium heat until the eggs have firmly set and the cheese is melted, about 3 minutes. Serve immediately.

NUTRITION INFORMATION (PER SERVING):

Calories: 340   Fat: 23 g   Carbohydrate: 14 g   Protein: 22 g

---

Good for chewing and swallowing difficulties, constipation,
fatigue, loss of appetite, and weight gain.

Modification

If experiencing diarrhea or nausea and vomiting, omit the onion, garlic, green pepper, eggs, and cheese. Add 1 teaspoon each of onion powder and garlic powder, and 8 egg whites. Use spices as tolerated.

MODIFIED NUTRITION INFORMATION:

Calories: 130   Fat: 3 g   Carbohydrate: 11 g   Protein: 16 g

---

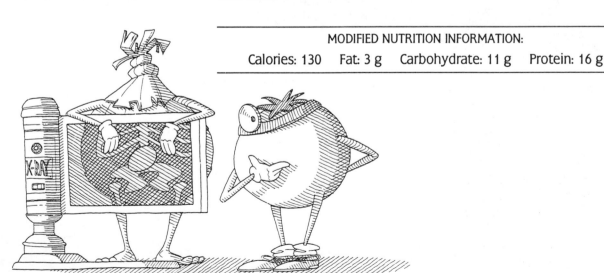

Mexican Scrambled Eggs

Yield: 1 serving
Preparation time: 20 minutes

2 eggs

1 tablespoon low-fat milk

¼ teaspoon salt

¼ cup chopped avocado

¼ cup kidney beans, cooked fresh or canned, rinsed and drained

½ teaspoon chili powder

1 tablespoon low-fat cottage cheese

1 slice whole grain bread, toasted

For a real Mexican flavor, try serving this dish with flour or corn tortillas instead of toast. If you are using dried beans, see page 212 for cooking instructions.

1. Place the eggs, milk, and salt in a small bowl, and beat with a wire whisk until frothy.

2. Pour the egg mixture into a frying pan coated with nonstick cooking spray over medium-high heat. Stir gently until the eggs are partially set, about 2 minutes.

3. Add the avocado and beans, and sprinkle with the chili powder. Continue to gently stir until the eggs are well set, about 2 minutes.

4. Spread the cottage cheese on the toasted bread. Place the eggs on top. Serve immediately.

NUTRITION INFORMATION (PER SERVING):

Calories: 380   Fat: 21 g   Carbohydrate: 29 g   Protein: 23 g

---

Good for alterations in taste, constipation, fatigue, and weight gain.

Modification

If experiencing chewing and swallowing difficulties or mouth and throat sores, omit the kidney beans, chili powder, and toasted bread. Use ¼ cup refried beans, and either untoasted bread or a flour tortilla.

MODIFIED NUTRITION INFORMATION:

Calories: 380   Fat: 21 g   Carbohydrate: 30 g   Protein: 23 g

---

Oven Omelet

Yield: 2 servings
Preparation time: 35 to 45 minutes

4 eggs

½ cup low-fat milk

¼ teaspoon salt

⅓ cup chopped corned beef or ham

½ cup grated cheese of your choice

1 teaspoon onion powder

This recipe is easy to prepare. Use any type of cheese you have on hand.

1. Preheat the oven to 325°F.

2. Place the eggs, milk, and salt in a small bowl, and beat with a wire whisk until frothy. Add the corned beef or ham, cheese, and onion powder, and mix thoroughly.

3. Coat an 8-inch square baking dish with nonstick cooking spray. Pour the egg mixture into the baking dish, and bake for 20 to 30 minutes, or until the eggs are well set. Serve immediately.

NUTRITION INFORMATION (PER SERVING):
Calories: 400   Fat: 27 g   Carbohydrate: 5 g   Protein: 33 g

Good for alterations in taste, chewing and swallowing difficulties, dry mouth, fatigue, mouth and throat sores, and weight gain.

Breakfast Sandwich

Yield: 4 sandwiches
Preparation time: 10 to 25 minutes

8 frozen waffles

¼ cup peanut butter

2 ripe bananas, sliced

¼ cup strawberry jam

This is an easy-to-make sandwich that can be made ahead of time, wrapped in foil, and frozen. To thaw a frozen sandwich, place in an oven preheated to 350°F for about 20 minutes, or until heated thoroughly.

1. Heat the waffles in a toaster, microwave, oven, or frying pan.

2. Spread the peanut butter on four of the waffles. Place the banana slices on the peanut butter.

3. Spread the jam on the remaining four waffles. Place the jam-spread waffles on top of the peanut butter-spread waffles. Serve immediately, or freeze.

NUTRITION INFORMATION (PER SANDWICH):
Calories: 405   Fat: 15 g   Carbohydrate: 62 g   Protein: 9 g

Good for fatigue and weight gain.

Scrambled Eggs With Herbs

Yield: 3 servings
Preparation time: 15 minutes

6 eggs

¼ cup water

2 tablespoons low-fat milk

¼ teaspoon salt

¼ teaspoon black pepper

¼ teaspoon dried dill, or ¼ tablespoon chopped fresh

¼ teaspoon dried oregano, or ¼ tablespoon chopped fresh

These eggs taste great when fresh herbs are used, but are also delicious with dried herbs. Instead of toast, try serving this dish with orzo—a type of pasta that looks like rice. Or accompany it with tortellini.

1. Coat an 8-inch frying pan with nonstick cooking spray, and preheat over medium heat.

2. Place all the ingredients in a medium-sized bowl, and beat with a wire whisk until frothy.

3. Pour the egg mixture into the frying pan, stirring gently to scramble, until the eggs are very firm, about 5 minutes. Serve immediately.

NUTRITION INFORMATION (PER SERVING):

Calories: 155   Fat: 10 g   Carbohydrate: 2 g   Protein: 13 g

---

Good for alterations in taste, chewing and swallowing difficulties,
dry mouth, fatigue, mouth and throat sores,
nausea and vomiting, and weight gain.

Modification

If experiencing diarrhea, omit the eggs, and use 3 eggs and 6 egg whites. Omit the low-fat milk, and use 2 tablespoons light soymilk or lactose-reduced milk.

MODIFIED NUTRITION INFORMATION:

Calories: 110   Fat: 5 g   Carbohydrate: 2 g   Protein: 13 g

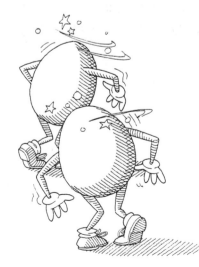

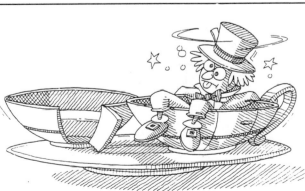

Scrambled Tofu

Yield: 3 servings
Preparation time: 15 to 20 minutes

1 teaspoon olive oil

1 clove garlic, minced

⅓ cup chopped onion

1 green bell pepper, seeded and chopped

½ cup sliced well-washed mushrooms

1 ¼ cups light tofu, drained

1 tablespoon soy sauce

This is a tasty alternative to scrambled eggs. It makes a great breakfast with fresh fruit and thick slices of a hearty, whole grain bread.

1. Place the oil in a medium-sized saucepan over medium-high heat. Add the garlic, onion, pepper, and mushrooms, and sauté until tender, about 3 minutes.

2. Add the tofu, and cook for 10 to 15 minutes, or until the water has boiled off.

3. Add the soy sauce right before serving. Serve immediately.

NUTRITION INFORMATION (PER SERVING):
Calories: 160   Fat: 8 g   Carbohydrate: 8 g   Protein: 16 g

Good for alterations in taste, chewing and swallowing difficulties, dry mouth, loss of appetite, and weight gain.

Modification

If experiencing diarrhea, omit the garlic, onion, and pepper. Use ½ tablespoon each garlic powder and onion powder, and 1 cup sliced mushrooms.

MODIFIED NUTRITION INFORMATION:
Calories: 130   Fat: 5 g   Carbohydrate: 7 g   Protein: 16 g

Buckwheat Pancakes

Yield: 6 pancakes
Preparation time: 30 minutes

2 tablespoons plain low-fat
  yogurt

1 cup low-fat milk

1 tablespoon molasses

1 tablespoon maple syrup

½ teaspoon vanilla extract

1 egg

1 cup buckwheat flour

1 teaspoon baking soda

Either you love buckwheat or you don't. Its flavor is the strongest of any of the grains, and its color the darkest. It is a rich source of fiber and B vitamins. You can make these pancakes ahead of time, wrap them in freezer-safe plastic wrap, and freeze them for 3 months. When you're ready for a quick breakfast, pop them in the toaster oven.

1. Coat a griddle or frying pan with nonstick cooking spray. Preheat over medium-high heat.

2. Place the yogurt, milk, molasses, maple syrup, vanilla, and egg in a medium-sized mixing bowl, and beat together with a wire whisk until smooth.

3. Place the flour and baking soda in a small bowl, and mix thoroughly. Add the egg mixture to the flour mixture, and whisk until smooth.

4. Pour ¼ cup batter per pancake onto the griddle or frying pan. When the pancakes are covered in bubbles, flip them over. Cook until well done, about 3 minutes. Serve immediately with your favorite topping.

NUTRITION INFORMATION (PER 2-PANCAKE SERVING, WITHOUT TOPPING):
Calories: 220   Fat: 5 g   Carbohydrate: 37 g   Protein: 9 g

Good for constipation, fatigue, loss of appetite,
nausea and vomiting, and weight gain.

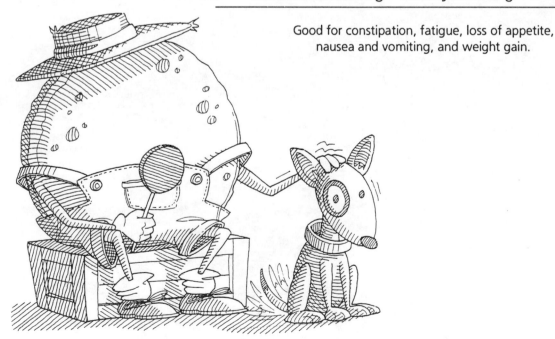

Cottage Cheese Pancakes

Yield: 4 pancakes
Preparation time: 35 minutes

1 cup low-fat cottage cheese

2 eggs

2 tablespoons whole wheat flour

¼ cup wheat germ

1 tablespoon butter

1 cup unsweetened applesauce

2 teaspoons ground cinnamon

The cottage cheese serves to boost the protein level in these fiber-rich pancakes. Make them in advance, wrap them in freezer-safe plastic wrap, and freeze for up to 3 months. Reheat in either the oven or the toaster oven.

1. Coat a griddle or frying pan with nonstick cooking spray. Preheat over medium-high heat.

2. Place the cottage cheese, eggs, flour, wheat germ, and butter in a medium-sized bowl, and mix thoroughly.

3. Pour ½ cup batter per pancake onto the griddle or frying pan. When the pancakes are covered in bubbles, flip them over. Cook until well done, about 3 minutes.

4. Top the pancakes with the applesauce, and sprinkle with the cinnamon. Serve immediately.

NUTRITION INFORMATION (PER 2-PANCAKE SERVING):

Calories: 365   Fat: 14 g   Carbohydrate: 34 g   Protein: 26 g

---

Good for chewing and swallowing difficulties, constipation, dry mouth, fatigue, mouth and throat sores, and weight gain.

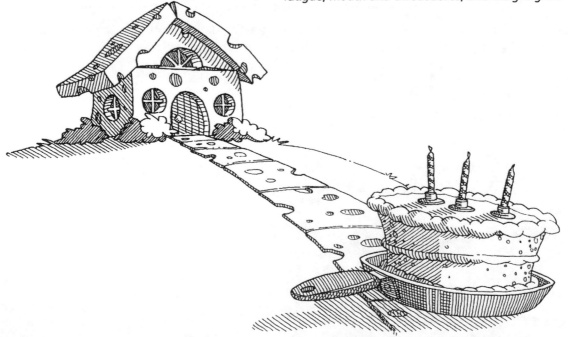

Lactose-Free Peach Pancakes

Yield: 2 pancakes
Preparation time: 30 minutes

½ cup cold water

1 teaspoon vanilla extract

1 teaspoon lemon juice

8 egg whites

¼ cup plus 3 tablespoons apple juice, divided

1 cup white flour

1 teaspoon baking powder

1 tablespoon ground cinnamon

2 well-washed peaches, peeled and sliced

These delicious pancakes are made without milk, so that even if you don't tolerate dairy products, you can still enjoy a wonderful pancake breakfast.

1. Coat a 6-inch frying pan with nonstick cooking spray, and preheat over medium heat. Preheat the oven to 400°F.

2. Place the water, vanilla, lemon juice, egg whites, and 3 tablespoons of the apple juice in a large bowl, and mix thoroughly. Place the flour and baking powder in another bowl, and mix thoroughly. Add the egg mixture to the flour mixture, and stir until smooth.

3. Place the remaining ¼ cup apple juice and 1 teaspoon of the cinnamon in the frying pan. Add the peach slices, and sauté until golden brown. Remove half of the peaches from the pan.

4. Pour half of the pancake batter over the remaining peaches, and cook on one side until set, about 2 minutes. Then, carefully slide the pancake onto a large plate, hold the frying pan over the pancake, and lay the pancake back into the frying pan, batter side down. Cook the other side until set.

5. Slide the pancake into a nonstick baking dish, and set aside. Make the second pancake, and slide it into the baking dish.

6. Sprinkle the pancakes with the remaining cinnamon, and bake at 400°F for 5 minutes. Serve immediately.

NUTRITION INFORMATION (PER 1-PANCAKE SERVING):

Calories: 390   Fat: 2 g   Carbohydrate: 74 g   Protein: 23 g

---

Good for alterations in taste, chewing and swallowing difficulties, diarrhea, dry mouth, loss of appetite, mouth and throat sores, and nausea and vomiting.

Oatmeal Pancakes

Yield: 8 pancakes
Preparation time: 25 minutes

1 cup white flour

½ cup quick-cooking oats

1 teaspoon baking powder

½ teaspoon salt

1 tablespoon canola oil

1 cup low-fat milk

2 egg whites

These pancakes are a real treat when topped with warmed applesauce or apple-cinnamon yogurt.

1. Coat a griddle or frying pan with nonstick cooking spray. Preheat over medium-high heat.

2. Place the flour, oats, baking powder, and salt in a medium-sized bowl, and mix thoroughly. Add the oil, milk, and egg whites, and stir until just moistened.

3. Pour ¼ cup batter per pancake onto the griddle. When the pancakes are covered in bubbles, flip them over. Cook until well done, about 3 minutes. Serve immediately with your favorite topping.

NUTRITION INFORMATION (PER 2-PANCAKE SERVING, WITHOUT TOPPING):
Calories: 220   Fat: 6 g   Carbohydrate: 34 g   Protein: 9 g

Good for chewing and swallowing difficulties, dry mouth,
fatigue, loss of appetite, mouth and throat sores,
nausea and vomiting, and weight gain.

Modification

If experiencing diarrhea, omit the low-fat milk, and use 1 cup light soymilk or lactose-reduced milk.

MODIFIED NUTRITION INFORMATION:
Calories: 190   Fat: 4 g   Carbohydrate: 31 g   Protein: 7 g

Orangy French Toast

Yield: 12 pieces
Preparation time: 25 minutes

6 eggs

⅔ cup orange juice

⅓ cup low-fat milk

3 tablespoons sugar

1 teaspoon vanilla extract

¼ teaspoon salt

½ teaspoon ground cinnamon

½ teaspoon ground nutmeg

12 slices whole wheat bread

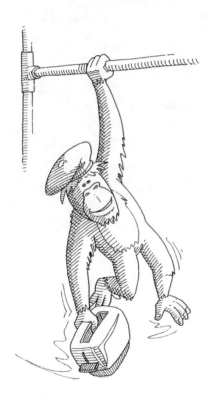

Our favorite toppings for this French toast are cinnamon and yogurt.

1. Coat a griddle or frying pan with nonstick cooking spray. Preheat over medium-high heat.

2. Place all the ingredients except the bread in a medium-sized bowl, and beat together until thoroughly mixed. Dip a slice of the bread into mixture, coating all sides, and soak for 30 seconds.

3. Place the bread on the griddle, and cook until well browned and the egg mixture is set. Flip the bread and cook the other side. Repeat until all the bread is used. Serve immediately with your favorite topping.

NUTRITION INFORMATION (PER 3-PIECE SERVING, WITHOUT TOPPING):
Calories: 240   Fat: 7 g   Carbohydrate: 32 g   Protein: 11 g

---

Good for alterations in taste, chewing and swallowing difficulties, dry mouth, and weight gain.

Modification

If experiencing diarrhea or nausea and vomiting, omit the eggs, milk, and whole wheat bread, and use 12 egg whites, ⅓ cup either light soymilk or lactose-reduced milk, and 12 slices white bread.

MODIFIED NUTRITION INFORMATION:
Calories: 195   Fat: 2 g   Carbohydrate: 32 g   Protein: 11 g

---

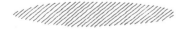

The Breadbasket

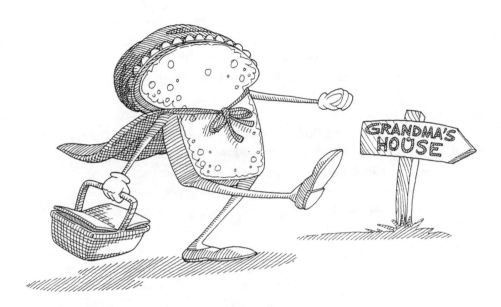

There is no smell quite as tempting as that of bread, muffins, or biscuits in the oven. In this chapter, we've provided recipes for breads that are quick to make and delicious to eat. You will find a range of tastes, from the sweet Jam-Stuffed Biscuits to the flavorful Herb Bread.

Bread is a nutritious addition to any meal, and makes a good choice for snacking. It is high in complex carbohydrates and easy to digest. We've chosen recipes that are generally low in fat. In several recipes, we've substituted applesauce for oil to create moist and tasty low-fat treats—these are also the breads to try if you have trouble chewing and swallowing. To boost the calories of bread, top it with peanut butter, low-fat cottage cheese, fruit spreads, sliced cheese, or low-fat hummus.

You can make the breads in this section ahead of time and freeze them for up to three months. This is an especially good idea if you are fatigued—prepare the breads when your energy level is up, or ask someone to help you. To ensure freshness and avoid mold, store bread in an airtight container, or wrap it tightly in foil or plastic. Breads can be stored at room temperature or in the refrigerator. Do not eat bread with visible mold spots. If mold is present, throw out the entire loaf.

Recipe-by-Symptoms Chart

Different recipes in this section are designed to address different symptoms that commonly occur in people with HIV disease. This chart can help you find recipes to help ease your symptoms. You'll note that some recipes address multiple symptoms.

ALTERATIONS IN TASTE	Apricot Bread, Cranberry Bread, Ham and Cheese Biscuits, Lemon Yogurt Muffins, Microwave Bran Muffins, Pumpkin Raisin Muffins, Strawberry Muffins, Sweet Potato Biscuits, Sweet Potato Muffins, Tangy Orange Bread
CHEWING AND SWALLOWING DIFFICULTIES	California Corn Bread, Cranberry Bread, Herb Bread, Lemon Yogurt Muffins, Low-Fat Banana Bread, Microwave Bran Muffins, Strawberry Muffins, Sweet Potato Biscuits, Zucchini Bread
CONSTIPATION	Apricot Bread, Herb Bread, Microwave Bran Muffins, Prune Muffins, Sweet Potato Muffins, Zucchini Bread
DIARRHEA	Banana English Muffin, California Corn Bread, Herb Bread (modified), Lemon Yogurt Muffins (modified), Low-Fat Banana Bread, Pumpkin Raisin Muffins (modified), Strawberry Muffins (modified), Tangy Orange Bread, Zucchini Bread (modified)
DRY MOUTH	Cranberry Bread, Lemon Yogurt Muffins, Low-Fat Banana Bread
FATIGUE	All (make a double batch when feeling well, and store in freezer for up to three months)
LOSS OF APPETITE	Apricot Bread, Banana English Muffin, California Corn Bread, Cranberry Bread, Ham and Cheese Biscuits, Herb Bread, Lemon Yogurt Muffins, Low-Fat Banana Bread, Microwave Bran Muffins, Prune Muffins, Pumpkin Raisin Muffins, Strawberry Muffins, Sweet Potato Biscuits, Sweet Potato Muffins, Zucchini Bread
MOUTH AND THROAT SORES	Low-Fat Banana Bread, Microwave Bran Muffins, Strawberry Muffins, Sweet Potato Biscuits, Zucchini Bread

NAUSEA AND VOMITING	Banana English Muffin, California Corn Bread, Cranberry Bread, Herb Bread, Lemon Yogurt Muffins, Low-Fat Banana Bread, Microwave Bran Muffins, Pumpkin Raisin Muffins, Strawberry Muffins, Sweet Potato Biscuits, Tangy Orange Bread
WEIGHT GAIN	Apricot Bread, Banana English Muffin, California Corn Bread, Ham and Cheese Biscuits, Herb Bread, Jam-Stuffed Biscuits, Lemon Yogurt Muffins, Prune Muffins, Pumpkin Raisin Muffins, Strawberry Muffins, Sweet Potato Biscuits, Sweet Potato Muffins, Tangy Orange Bread, Zucchini Bread

California Corn Bread

Yield: 6 servings
Preparation time: 10 minutes to assemble; 20 minutes to bake

1 cup cornmeal

1 cup white flour

¼ cup sugar

4 teaspoons baking powder

¼ teaspoon salt

1 cup light soymilk

3 egg whites, lightly beaten

¼ cup unsweetened applesauce

This corn bread is unique in that applesauce is used in place of the oil normally used. This gives the bread a moist texture with less fat than most corn breads. It's delicious.

1. Preheat the oven to 425°F.

2. Place the cornmeal, flour, sugar, baking powder, and salt in a medium-sized bowl, and mix thoroughly. Add the soymilk, egg whites, and applesauce, and mix thoroughly.

3. Coat an 8-inch square baking pan with nonstick cooking spray. Spread the mixture evenly in the pan, and bake for 20 minutes, or until the bread is firm. Let the bread stand in the pan for 5 minutes, then remove and place on a wire rack to cool.

NUTRITION INFORMATION (PER SERVING):
Calories: 230   Fat: 1 g   Carbohydrate: 49 g   Protein: 7 g

Good for chewing and swallowing difficulties, diarrhea, fatigue, loss of appetite, nausea and vomiting, and weight gain.

Apricot Bread

Yield: 12 ½-inch slices
Preparation time: 15 minutes to assemble; 45 minutes to bake

½ pound dried apricots, chopped

1 ½ cups orange juice

1 cup low-fat milk

¼ cup canola oil

¼ cup honey

2 ½ teaspoons baking powder

2 ½ cups whole wheat flour

½ cup chopped walnuts

This sweet bread makes a delicious snack or dessert. To boost the calorie count, try topping it with low-fat cream cheese.

1. Preheat the oven to 350°F.

2. Place the apricots and orange juice in a small saucepan over low heat. Cook until the juice is absorbed, and the apricots are soft and mushy—about 5 minutes. Set aside.

3. Place the milk, oil, and honey in a medium-sized bowl, and beat together until smooth. Place the baking powder and flour in a separate bowl, and mix thoroughly. Add the milk mixture to the flour mixture while stirring slowly with a spoon. Add the apricots and nuts, and mix thoroughly.

4. Coat an 8-x-4-inch loaf pan with nonstick cooking spray, then dust with flour. Spread the batter evenly in the loaf pan. Bake for 45 minutes, or until the loaf is firm to the touch—an inserted knife or toothpick should come out clean. Let the loaf stand in the pan for 5 minutes, then remove and place on a wire rack to cool.

NUTRITION INFORMATION (PER 1-SLICE SERVING):
Calories: 370   Fat: 13 g   Carbohydrate: 60 g   Protein: 9 g

Good for alterations in taste, constipation, fatigue, loss of appetite, and weight gain.

Cranberry Bread

*Yield: 12 ½-inch slices
Preparation time: 15 minutes to assemble; 65 minutes to bake*

1 ¾ cups white flour

1 teaspoon baking soda

1 cup sugar

1 teaspoon salt

¾ cup unsweetened applesauce

2 egg whites

1 teaspoon vanilla extract

1 cup cranberries, well-washed fresh or thawed frozen

This fragrant bread is tasty and tart, but not too sweet.

1. Preheat the oven to 350°F.

2. Place the flour, baking soda, sugar, and salt in a medium-sized bowl, and mix thoroughly. Place the applesauce, egg whites, and vanilla in a separate bowl, and beat together until smooth. Add the applesauce mixture to the flour mixture, and stir until the dry ingredients are just moistened. Fold in the cranberries.

3. Coat an 8-x-4-inch loaf pan with nonstick cooking spray, then dust with flour. Spread the batter evenly in the loaf pan. Bake for 65 minutes, or until the loaf is firm to the touch—an inserted knife or toothpick should come out clean. Let the loaf stand in the pan for 5 minutes, then remove and place on a wire rack to cool.

NUTRITION INFORMATION (PER 1-SLICE SERVING):
Calories: 145   Fat: less than 1 g   Carbohydrate: 34 g   Protein: 3 g

Good for alterations in taste, chewing and swallowing difficulties, dry mouth, fatigue, loss of appetite, and nausea and vomiting.

Herb Bread

Yield: 12 ½-inch slices
Preparation time: 15 minutes
to assemble; 50 to 55 minutes
to bake

1 ½ cups whole wheat flour

1 ½ cups white flour

2 tablespoons sugar

1 tablespoon baking powder

¼ teaspoon ground nutmeg

1 ½ teaspoons dried thyme,
   rosemary, oregano, or basil

½ teaspoon salt

1 egg, beaten

1 ½ cups low-fat milk

2 tablespoons canola oil

This bread is very tasty and so easy to make. It goes great with bean dishes, soups, pasta, and stews, and can be used for sandwiches. Instead of using only thyme, rosemary, oregano, or basil, feel free to use any combination of these herbs that you like.

1. Preheat the oven to 350°F.

2. Place the flours, sugar, baking powder, nutmeg, herbs, and salt in a large bowl, and mix thoroughly. Place the egg, milk, and oil in a separate bowl, and beat together thoroughly. Add the egg mixture to the flour mixture, and stir until the dry ingredients are just moistened.

3. Coat an 8-x-4-inch loaf pan with nonstick cooking spray, then dust with flour. Spread the batter in the loaf pan. Bake for 50 to 55 minutes, or until the loaf is firm to the touch—an inserted knife or toothpick should come out clean. Let the loaf stand in the pan for 5 minutes, then remove and place on a wire rack to cool.

NUTRITION INFORMATION (PER 1-SLICE SERVING):
Calories: 160   Fat: 4 g   Carbohydrate: 27 g   Protein: 5 g

Good for chewing and swallowing difficulties, constipation, fatigue, loss of appetite, nausea and vomiting, and weight gain.

Modification

If experiencing diarrhea, omit the egg and milk, and use 2 egg whites and 1 ½ cups light soymilk or lactose-reduced milk. Omit the whole wheat flour, and use 3 cups white flour.

MODIFIED NUTRITION INFORMATION:
Calories: 160   Fat: 3 g   Carbohydrate: 28 g   Protein: 4 g

Low-Fat Banana Bread

*Yield: 12 ½-inch slices
Preparation time: 15 minutes to
assemble; 60 minutes to bake*

½ cup unsweetened
  applesauce

½ cup sugar

2 tablespoons canola oil

4 egg whites, lightly beaten

1 cup mashed banana (2 large,
  ripe bananas)

1 teaspoon lemon juice

2 cups white flour

1 tablespoon baking powder

½ teaspoon salt

This bread is a delicious way to use up your extra-ripe bananas. Try warming it up and topping it with peanut butter for a calorie-rich treat.

1. Preheat the oven to 375°F.

2. Place the applesauce, sugar, and oil in a medium-sized bowl, and mix thoroughly. Stir in the egg whites. Place the banana and lemon juice in a separate bowl, and mix thoroughly. Add to the applesauce mixture.

3. Place the flour, baking powder, and salt in separate bowl, and mix thoroughly. Slowly stir the applesauce mixture into the flour mixture until the dry ingredients are just moistened.

4. Coat an 8-x-4-inch loaf pan with nonstick cooking spray, then dust with flour. Spread the batter evenly in the loaf pan. Bake for 60 minutes, or until the loaf is firm to the touch—an inserted knife or toothpick should come out clean. Let the loaf stand in the pan for 5 minutes, then remove and place on a wire rack to cool.

NUTRITION INFORMATION (PER 1-SLICE SERVING):
Calories: 155   Fat: 2 g   Carbohydrate: 30 g   Protein: 4 g

Good for chewing and swallowing difficulties, diarrhea,
dry mouth, fatigue, loss of appetite, mouth and throat sores,
and nausea and vomiting.

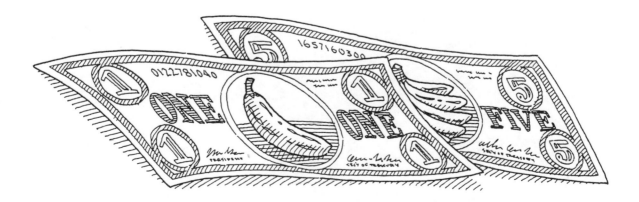

Tangy Orange Bread

Yield: 12 ¹/₂-inch slices
Preparation time: 15 minutes to assemble; 60 minutes to bake

1 ½ cups white flour

½ cup sugar

2 teaspoons baking powder

½ teaspoon salt

¼ cup unsweetened applesauce

4 egg whites

½ cup orange juice

GLAZE

¼ cup plus 2 tablespoons powdered sugar

1 ½ tablespoons orange juice

This tangy, tart, and not-too-sweet bread is low in fat. But don't let that dissuade you from serving it for dessert!

1. Preheat the oven to 325°F.

2. Place the flour, sugar, baking powder, and salt in a large bowl, and mix thoroughly. Place the applesauce, egg whites, and orange juice in a separate bowl, and mix thoroughly. Add the applesauce mixture to the flour mixture, and stir until the dry ingredients are just moistened.

3. Coat an 8-x-4-inch loaf pan with nonstick cooking spray, then dust with flour. Spread the batter evenly in the loaf pan. Bake for 60 minutes, or until the loaf is firm to the touch—an inserted knife or toothpick should come out clean. Let the loaf stand in the pan for 5 minutes, then remove and place on a wire rack to cool.

4. While the bread is cooling, prepare the glaze by placing the powdered sugar and orange juice in a small bowl, and stirring until thoroughly mixed. Place the cooled bread on a plate, and drizzle with the glaze.

NUTRITION INFORMATION (PER 1-SLICE SERVING):

Calories: 170   Fat: less than 1 g   Carbohydrate: 38 g   Protein: 4 g

Good for alterations in taste, diarrhea, fatigue,
nausea and vomiting, and weight gain.

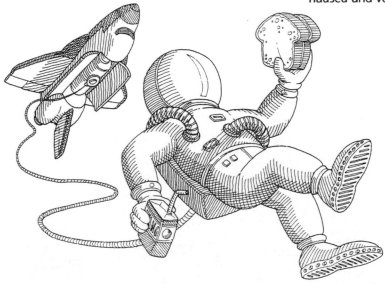

Zucchini Bread

Yield: 12 ½-inch slices
Preparation time: 15 minutes to assemble; 50 minutes to bake

1 cup sugar

¾ cup unsweetened applesauce

1 cup whole wheat flour

½ cup white flour

1 teaspoon baking powder

1 teaspoon baking soda

1 teaspoon salt

1 teaspoon ground cinnamon

1 cup grated well-washed zucchini (2 or 3 zucchini)

1 teaspoon vanilla extract

2 eggs, lightly beaten

This tasty bread makes a hearty snack. Try topping it with plain or vanilla low-fat yogurt, or with low-fat cream cheese.

1. Preheat the oven to 350°F.

2. Place the sugar and applesauce in a medium-sized bowl, and mix until smooth. Place the flours, baking powder, baking soda, salt, and cinnamon in a separate bowl, and mix thoroughly. Add the applesauce mixture to the flour mixture, and stir until mixed. Add the zucchini, vanilla, and eggs, and mix thoroughly.

3. Coat an 8-x-4-inch loaf pan with nonstick cooking spray, then dust with flour. Spread the batter evenly in the loaf pan. Bake for 50 minutes, or until the loaf is firm to the touch and an inserted knife or toothpick comes out clean. Let the loaf stand in the pan for for 5 minutes, then remove and place on a wire rack for cooling.

NUTRITION INFORMATION (PER 1-SLICE SERVING):

Calories: 160   Fat: 3 g   Carbohydrate: 31 g   Protein: 4 g

Good for chewing and swallowing difficulties, constipation, fatigue, loss of appetite, mouth and throat sores, and weight gain.

Modification

If experiencing diarrhea, omit the whole wheat flour, and use 1 ½ cups white flour. The nutrition information doesn't change.

Jam-Stuffed Biscuits

Yield: 8 biscuits
Preparation time: 10 minutes
to assemble; 12 to 15 minutes
to bake

1 8-ounce package refrigerated
biscuits

½ cup jam, any flavor

¼ cup low-fat milk

2 tablespoons sugar

These easy-to-prepare biscuits make mouth-watering snacks or sweet additions to the breakfast table.

1. Preheat the oven to 375°F.

2. Separate the biscuits, and flatten them with a fork to twice their original size.

3. Place a heaping teaspoonful of jam in the center of each biscuit. Fold the biscuit over the jam, and seal the edges with a fork. Brush the biscuits with the milk, and sprinkle with the sugar.

4. Coat a cookie sheet with nonstick cooking spray. Place the biscuits on the sheet, and bake for 12 to 15 minutes, or until lightly golden brown. Immediately transfer to a wire rack to cool for about 5 minutes before serving.

NUTRITION INFORMATION (PER BISCUIT):
Calories: 170   Fat: 5 g   Carbohydrate: 30 g   Protein: 2 g

Good for fatigue and weight gain.

Ham and Cheese Biscuits

Yield: 12 biscuits
Preparation time: 10 minutes
to assemble; 20 to 25 minutes
to bake

1 ½ cups diced lean ham

2 cups white flour

1 cup shredded cheddar cheese

2 teaspoons baking powder

¼ teaspoon dried red pepper

1 cup low-fat milk

These high-protein biscuits make a hearty breakfast. Or serve them with a bowl of soup for a tasty dinner.

1. Preheat the oven to 400°F.

2. Coat a frying pan with nonstick cooking spray. Place the ham in the pan over medium heat, and sauté until hot, about 3 minutes.

3. Place the flour, cheese, baking powder, and red pepper in a large bowl, and mix thoroughly. Add the ham, and stir well. Add the milk, and stir until the dry ingredients are just moistened.

4. Coat a cookie sheet with nonstick cooking spray. Drop the dough by heaping tablespoonfuls onto the sheet, dividing the dough into 12 equal parts. Bake for 20 to 25 minutes, or until biscuits are lightly golden brown. Immediately transfer to a wire rack to cool for about 5 minutes before serving.

NUTRITION INFORMATION (PER BISCUIT):

Calories: 150   Fat: 5 g   Carbohydrate: 18 g   Protein: 9 g

Good for alterations in taste, fatigue,
loss of appetite, and weight gain.

Sweet Potato Biscuits

*Yield: 12 biscuits
Preparation time: 25 minutes to
assemble; 15 minutes to bake*

2 ⅔ cups white flour

2 tablespoons brown sugar,
  firmly packed

1 tablespoon baking powder

¼ teaspoon salt

3 tablespoons plus 1 teaspoon
  butter

¾ cup low-fat milk

1 cup mashed sweet potato,
  cooked fresh or canned

*These biscuits can easily be made ahead of time and frozen. Make sure to
wrap them tightly to avoid freezer burn.*

1. Preheat the oven to 450°F.

2. Place the flour, sugar, baking powder, and salt in a large bowl, and
mix thoroughly. Cut in the butter with either a pastry blender or two knives
until the mixture resembles coarse meal. Add the milk and sweet potato,
and stir until the dry ingredients are just moistened.

3. Turn the dough onto a floured surface, and knead it 4 or 5 times.
Flour a rolling pin and roll the dough to a ½-inch thickness. Cut the dough
with either a biscuit cutter or the rim of a glass—each biscuit should be
about 3 inches across.

4. Coat a cookie sheet with nonstick cooking spray. Place the biscuits
on the cookie sheet and bake for 15 minutes, or until lightly golden brown.
Immediately transfer to a wire rack to cool for about 5 minutes.

NUTRITION INFORMATION (PER BISCUIT):

Calories: 105   Fat: 2 g   Carbohydrate: 19 g   Protein: 2 g

Good for alterations in taste, chewing and swallowing difficulties,
loss of appetite, mouth and throat sores,
nausea and vomiting, and weight gain.

Banana English Muffin

Yield: 1 serving
Preparation time: 10 minutes

1 English muffin, sliced in half

1 ripe banana

1 teaspoon honey

½ teaspoon ground cinnamon

This muffin is easy to make, tasty, and full of energy nutrients.

1. Toast the English muffin. While the muffin is toasting, slice the banana.

2. Arrange the banana slices on the toasted muffin. Drizzle with the honey and sprinkle with the cinnamon.

3. Place the muffin under the broiler or in a toaster oven, and broil until the tops are browned—about 3 minutes.

NUTRITION INFORMATION (PER SERVING):
Calories: 350   Fat: 2 g   Carbohydrate: 75 g   Protein: 7 g

Good for diarrhea, fatigue, loss of appetite,
nausea and vomiting, and weight gain.

Microwave Bran Muffins

Yield: 4 muffins
Preparation time: 15 to 20 minutes

1 cup water

3 cups bran cereal

½ cup butter

1 ½ cups sugar

2 eggs

1 ½ cups white flour

1 cup whole wheat flour

2 teaspoons baking soda

2 cups buttermilk (see "Buttermilk Substitute")

You want hot, fresh bran muffins for breakfast, but you're always in a hurry? No problem! These microwave muffins can be made in minutes, since the batter can be kept in the refrigerator. Also, this recipe can easily be cut in half. If you do not have custard cups or a muffin tin, use a small, shallow bowl or a coffee cup.

1. Boil the water.

2. Place the bran cereal in a large, covered storage container. Stir in the water until the cereal is just moistened.

3. Cut the butter into chunks, and add to the hot cereal. Stir to cover the butter, and set aside until the butter softens, about 3 minutes.

4. Stir in the sugar and eggs, and beat well. Stir in the flours, baking soda, and buttermilk, and mix thoroughly.

5. Spray the custard cups or muffin tin with nonstick cooking spray. Prepare from 1 to 4 cups, depending on the number of muffins desired. Spoon the batter into the cups until the cups are half full. Cook the muffins, uncovered, on high power until no doughy spots remain:

1 muffin—1 to 1 $\frac{1}{2}$ minutes
2 muffins—1 $\frac{1}{2}$ to 2 minutes
4 muffins—2 to 2 $\frac{1}{2}$ minutes

6. Serve immediately. Store the remaining batter in an airtight container in the refrigerator for up to 4 weeks.

NUTRITION INFORMATION (PER MUFFIN):

Calories: 100   Fat: 3 g   Carbohydrate: 18 g   Protein: 2 g

Good for alterations in taste, chewing and swallowing difficulties, constipation, fatigue, loss of appetite, mouth and throat sores, and nausea and vomiting.

Buttermilk Substitute

If you don't have buttermilk, you can make an acceptable substitute. For every $\frac{1}{2}$ cup of buttermilk called for in the recipe, use $\frac{1}{2}$ cup of low-fat milk to which 1 $\frac{1}{2}$ teaspoons vinegar has been added.

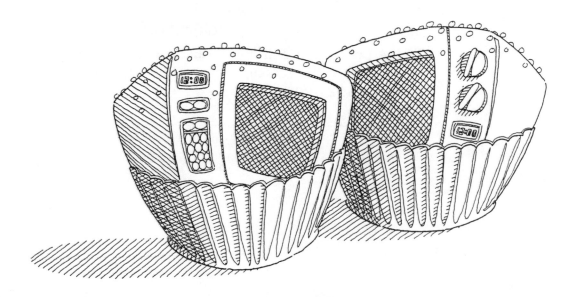

Lemon Yogurt Muffins

*Yield: 12 muffins
Preparation time: 15 minutes
to assemble; 18 to 20 minutes
to bake*

¼ cup plus 2 tablespoons
　honey

¼ cup butter

1 cup plain low-fat yogurt

1 egg

¼ cup lemon juice, preferably
　fresh-squeezed

½ teaspoon freshly grated
　lemon peel

1 cup white flour

1 cup whole wheat flour

¼ teaspoon ground nutmeg

1 ½ teaspoons baking soda

¼ teaspoon salt

Serve these muffins with a soothing cup of herbal tea.

1. Preheat the oven to 375°F.

2. Place the honey and butter in a small saucepan over low heat, and cook until they melt together, about 5 minutes. In the meantime, place the yogurt, egg, lemon juice, and lemon peel in a medium-sized bowl, and beat together until thoroughly mixed. Remove the honey mixture from the heat, and add to the yogurt mixture. Mix thoroughly.

3. Sift the dry ingredients together into a separate bowl. Add the wet ingredients, and stir until the dry ingredients are just moistened.

4. Coat muffin cups with nonstick cooking spray, and fill two-thirds full with the batter. Bake for 18 to 20 minutes, or until firm to the touch. Let the muffins stand in the tin for 5 minutes, then remove and place on a wire rack to cool.

NUTRITION INFORMATION (PER MUFFIN):

Calories: 155　　Fat: 4 g　　Carbohydrate: 25 g　　Protein: 4 g

Good for alterations in taste, chewing and swallowing difficulties,
dry mouth, fatigue, loss of appetite, nausea and vomiting,
and weight gain.

Modification

If experiencing diarrhea, omit the butter, yogurt, egg, and whole wheat flour. Use 1 ¼ cups unsweetened applesauce, 2 cups white flour, and 2 egg whites.

MODIFIED NUTRITION INFORMATION:

Calories: 125　　Fat: less than 1 g　　Carbohydrate: 28 g　　Protein: 3 g

---

Prune Muffins

Yield: 12 muffins
Preparation time: 15 minutes to assemble; 20 minutes to bake

¾ cup white flour

½ cup whole wheat flour

½ cup rolled oats

⅓ cup sugar

¼ cup cornmeal

¼ cup wheat germ

1 ½ teaspoons baking powder

½ teaspoon baking soda

1 teaspoon ground cinnamon

¼ teaspoon salt

1 cup chopped prunes

1 cup plain low-fat yogurt

3 tablespoons canola oil

1 egg, lightly beaten

The prunes give these mildly dense muffins a sweet flavor you'll enjoy. Prunes are a good source of iron, potassium, fiber, and calories.

1. Preheat the oven to 400°F.

2. Place the first ten ingredients in a large bowl, and mix thoroughly. Place the remaining ingredients in a separate bowl, and beat well with a wire whisk. Make a well in the center of the dry mixture, and add the wet mixture all at once, stirring until the dry ingredients are just moistened.

3. Coat muffin cups with nonstick cooking spray, and divide the batter evenly among the cups. Bake for 20 minutes, or until a knife or toothpick inserted into the center comes out clean. Remove the muffins from the pan immediately, and cool on a wire rack.

NUTRITION INFORMATION (PER MUFFIN):

Calories: 170   Fat: 5 g   Carbohydrate: 29 g   Protein: 5 g

Good for constipation, fatigue, loss of appetite, and weight gain.

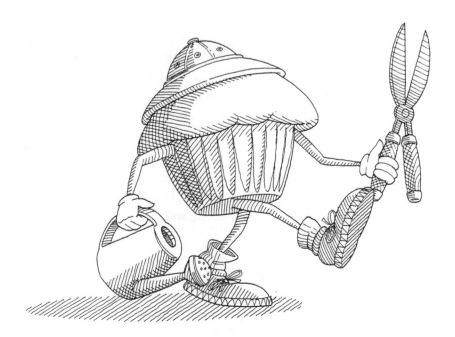

Pumpkin Raisin Muffins

Yield: 25 muffins
Preparation time: 15 minutes
to assemble; 30 to 35 minutes
to bake

2 cups canned pumpkin purée

1 ¼ cups honey

4 eggs

1 cup evaporated skim milk

1 cup water

1 tablespoon canola oil

1 tablespoon ground cinnamon

1 teaspoon ground nutmeg

1 teaspoon ground ginger

¼ teaspoon ground cloves

3 ⅓ cups whole wheat flour

1 tablespoon baking soda

2 teaspoons baking powder

1 cup raisins

These tempting muffins will give you a taste of the holidays at any time of the year.

1. Preheat the oven to 350°F.

2. Place the first 10 ingredients in a large bowl, and mix thoroughly. Place the remaining ingredients in a separate bowl, and mix thoroughly. Add the wet mixture all at once to the dry mixture, and stir gently until the dry ingredients are just moistened. Gently stir in the raisins.

3. Coat muffin cups with nonstick cooking spray, and fill two-thirds full with the batter. Bake for 30 to 35 minutes, or until a knife or toothpick inserted into the center comes out clean. Cool the muffins for 15 minutes before removing from the tin.

NUTRITION INFORMATION (PER MUFFIN):
Calories: 150   Fat: 1 g   Carbohydrate: 33 g   Protein: 5 g

Good for alterations in taste, fatigue, loss of appetite,
nausea and vomiting, and weight gain.

Variation

To make pumpkin raisin loaves, pour the batter into two 8-x-4-inch loaf pans, and bake 60 to 65 minutes, or until firm to the touch—a knife or toothpick inserted into the center should come out clean. Let the loaves stand in the pans for 15 minutes. Then remove and place on a wire rack to cool.

Modification

If experiencing diarrhea, omit the eggs, milk, whole wheat flour, and raisins. Use 8 egg whites, 1 cup light soymilk or lactose-reduced milk, and 3 ½ cups white flour.

MODIFIED NUTRITION INFORMATION:
Calories: 135   Fat: 1 g   Carbohydrate: 29 g   Protein: 3 g

Strawberry Muffins

Yield: 12 muffins
Preparation time: 15 minutes to assemble; 25 minutes to bake

2 ½ cups white flour

⅔ cup sugar

1 teaspoon baking soda

1 teaspoon ground cinnamon

½ teaspoon salt

1 ½ cups strawberries, well-washed fresh or thawed frozen

1 cup buttermilk (see page 103)

¼ cup butter, melted

1 ¼ teaspoons vanilla extract

1 egg plus 1 egg white

1 ½ tablespoons sugar

These muffins are yummy!

1. Preheat the oven to 350°F.

2. Place the flour, sugar, baking soda, cinnamon, and salt in large bowl, and mix thoroughly. Add the strawberries, and gently stir until just mixed.

3. Place the buttermilk, butter, vanilla, and eggs in a separate bowl, and mix thoroughly. Make a well in the center of the flour mixture, and add the buttermilk mixture all at once, stirring until the dry ingredients are just moistened.

4. Coat muffin cups with nonstick cooking spray, and divide the batter evenly among the cups. Sprinkle the sugar evenly over the muffins. Bake for 25 minutes, or until an inserted knife or toothpick comes out clean. Remove the muffins from the tin immediately, and let them cool on a wire rack.

NUTRITION INFORMATION (PER MUFFIN):

Calories: 210   Fat: 6 g   Carbohydrate: 35 g   Protein: 4 g

Good for alterations in taste, chewing and swallowing difficulties, fatigue, loss of appetite, mouth and throat sores, nausea and vomiting, and weight gain.

Modification

If experiencing diarrhea, omit the buttermilk, butter, and egg, and use 1 cup light soymilk or lactose-reduced milk, ¼ cup margarine, and 3 egg whites.

MODIFIED NUTRITION INFORMATION:

Calories: 200   Fat: 4 g   Carbohydrate: 35 g   Protein: 4 g

Sweet Potato Muffins

Yield: 12 muffins
Preparation time: 15 minutes
to assemble; 25 to 30 minutes
to bake

1 cup mashed sweet potato,
   cooked fresh or canned

⅓ cup molasses

½ cup low-fat milk

½ cup canola oil

1 egg

1 cup whole wheat flour

⅓ cup oat bran

2 teaspoons baking powder

1 ¼ teaspoons ground
   cinnamon

¼ teaspoon ground nutmeg

¼ cup raisins

¼ cup chopped walnuts

½ teaspoon salt

Keep a bunch of these muffins on hand to encourage healthy snacking. They are full of fiber, beta-carotene, calcium, and iron.

1. Preheat the oven to 350°F.

2. Place the sweet potato, molasses, milk, oil, and egg in a medium-sized bowl, and beat with a fork or a wire whisk until smooth.

3. Place the remaining ingredients in a separate bowl, and mix thoroughly. Mix the sweet potato mixture into the flour mixture until the dry ingredients are just moistened.

4. Coat muffin cups with nonstick cooking spray, and divide the batter evenly among the cups. Bake for 25 to 30 minutes, or until an inserted knife or toothpick comes out clean. Remove the muffins from the tin immediately, and let them cool on a wire rack.

NUTRITION INFORMATION (PER MUFFIN):

Calories: 200   Fat: 11 g   Carbohydrate: 23 g   Protein: 3 g

---

Good for alterations in taste, constipation, fatigue,
loss of appetite, and weight gain.

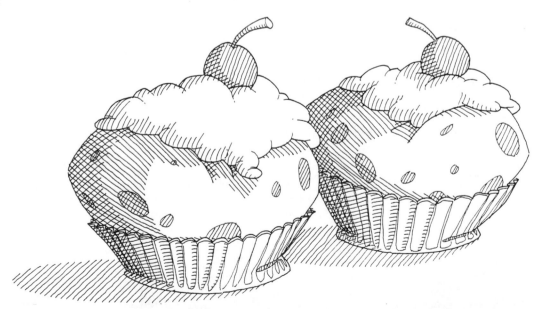

Blender Beverages

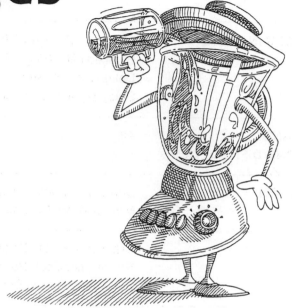

Blender beverages are a delicious and soothing way to boost your daily calorie and protein intake. Drink them with meals, or sip them throughout the day. You can store these drinks in the refrigerator, right in the blender container. Just be sure to finish a day's batch by the end of the day to avoid spoilage. You can freshen the drink by throwing in a few ice cubes and putting the container back on the blender for a few seconds.

These beverage recipes can be easily adjusted to meet your tolerances and tastes. Mix and match fruits to create your own recipes. To add carbohydrates, try using leftover rice or oatmeal. To boost protein, add tofu, creamy peanut butter, frozen pasteurized egg product, low-fat cottage cheese, or yogurt. For thicker smoothies, add more fruit and less liquid. If swallowing is a problem, adjust the amount of liquid used. You can also try adding flavorings such as cinnamon or vanilla before blending.

Obeying food safety rules is extremely important when making blender beverages. Remember to thoroughly wash or peel all fruits and vegetables prior to blending. Never use raw eggs. Raw eggs may carry salmonella and can make you very sick.

Recipe-by-Symptoms Chart

Different recipes in this section are designed to address different symptoms that commonly occur in people with HIV disease. This chart can help you find recipes to ease your symptoms. You'll note that some recipes address multiple symptoms.

ALTERATIONS IN TASTE	Blueberry Orange Whip, Cantaloupe Shake, Cranberry Punch, Fortified Milk, Ginger Punch, Lemon Blend, Orange Pineapple Delight, Peach Smoothie, Pear Icey, Raspberry Rice Smoothie, Spicy Squash Smoothie, Strawberry Delight
CHEWING AND SWALLOWING DIFFICULTIES	All
CONSTIPATION	Banana Oat Shake, Fortified Milk, Mid-Morning Pickup, Monster Mango Mash, Raspberry Rice Smoothie, Southern Buttermilk Cooler
DIARRHEA	Cranberry Punch, Fortified Milk, Ginger Punch, Honey Graham Shake (modified), Pear Icey, Spicy Squash Smoothie (modified), Strawberry Delight (modified)
DRY MOUTH	All
FATIGUE	Apple Pie à la Mode, Banana Oat Shake, Blueberry Orange Whip, Cantaloupe Shake, Carrot Shake, Cranberry Punch, Creamy Berry and Chocolate Shake, Fortified Milk, Fruit Salad Shake, Ginger Punch, Go Ape Shake, Honey Graham Shake, Mid-Morning Pickup, Monster Mango Mash, Nutty Whip, Peach Smoothie, Raspberry Rice Smoothie, Southern Buttermilk Cooler, Spicy Squash Smoothie, Strawberry Delight, Winter Warmer
LOSS OF APPETITE	Apple Pie à la Mode, Banana Oat Shake, Blueberry Orange Whip, Cantaloupe Shake, Cranberry Punch, Fortified Milk, Fruit Salad Shake, Ginger Punch, Go Ape Shake, Honey Graham Shake, Lemon Blend, Mid-Morning Pickup, Monster Mango Mash, Orange Pineapple Delight, Peach Smoothie, Pear Icey, Raspberry Rice Smoothie, Southern Buttermilk Cooler, Spicy Squash Smoothie, Strawberry Delight, Winter Warmer

MOUTH AND THROAT SORES	Apple Pie à la Mode, Banana Oat Shake, Cantaloupe Shake (modified), Carrot Shake, Creamy Berry and Chocolate Shake, Fortified Milk, Fruit Salad Shake, Go Ape Shake, Honey Graham Shake, Mid-Morning Pickup, Monster Mango Mash, Nutty Whip, Peach Smoothie, Raspberry Rice Smoothie, Southern Buttermilk Cooler, Spicy Squash Smoothie
NAUSEA AND VOMITING	Banana Oat Shake, Blueberry Orange Whip, Cantaloupe Shake, Carrot Shake, Cranberry Punch, Fortified Milk, Fruit Salad Shake, Ginger Punch, Lemon Blend, Monster Mango Mash, Orange Pineapple Delight, Peach Smoothie, Pear Icey, Raspberry Rice Smoothie, Southern Buttermilk Cooler, Spicy Squash Smoothie, Strawberry Delight
WEIGHT GAIN	Apple Pie à la Mode, Banana Oat Shake, Cantaloupe Shake, Carrot Shake, Creamy Berry and Chocolate Shake, Fortified Milk, Go Ape Shake, Honey Graham Shake, Lemon Blend, Mid-Morning Pickup, Nutty Whip, Orange Pineapple Delight, Peach Smoothie, Raspberry Rice Smoothie, Southern Buttermilk Cooler, Strawberry Delight, Winter Warmer

Apple Pie à la Mode

Yield: 1 serving
Preparation time: 10 minutes

1 cup canned apple pie filling

1 cup vanilla-flavored low-fat yogurt

½ cup low-fat milk

⅛ teaspoon ground cinnamon

If ice cream is too heavy, use nonfat frozen yogurt, low-fat cottage cheese, light tofu, or sherbet.

1. Put all the ingredients into a blender, and blend until smooth.

NUTRITION INFORMATION (PER SERVING):

Calories: 525   Fat: 5 g   Carbohydrate: 110 g   Protein: 14 g

---

Good for chewing and swallowing difficulties, dry mouth, fatigue, loss of appetite, mouth and throat sores, and weight gain.

Banana Oat Shake

Yield: 1 serving
Preparation time: 10 minutes

½ cup cooked oats (either quick-cooking or rolled), chilled

1 large ripe banana, sliced

⅔ cup low-fat milk

2 teaspoons brown sugar, firmly packed

1 teaspoon wheat germ

1 teaspoon vanilla extract

2 or 3 ice cubes

Oats, a high-energy food, is an excellent source of complex carbohydrates and soluble fiber.

1. Put all the ingredients into a blender, and blend until smooth.

NUTRITION INFORMATION (PER SERVING):

Calories: 330   Fat: 5 g   Carbohydrate: 63 g   Protein: 10 g

---

Good for chewing and swallowing difficulties, constipation, dry mouth, fatigue, loss of appetite, mouth and throat sores, nausea and vomiting, and weight gain.

Blueberry Orange Whip

Yield: 1 serving
Preparation time: 10 minutes

1 orange, peeled and sectioned

⅔ cup frozen blueberries

1 cup low-fat milk

¼ cup dry milk powder

Substitute fresh blueberries for frozen ones during berry season—May through September. Just remember to wash the berries very well right before using them, since blueberries washed before storage can develop mold. Fresh blueberries can be stored in the refrigerator for up to five days.

1. Put all the ingredients into a blender, and blend until smooth.

NUTRITION INFORMATION (PER SERVING):

Calories: 300   Fat: 6 g   Carbohydrate: 50 g   Protein: 16 g

---

Good for alterations in taste, chewing and swallowing difficulties, dry mouth, fatigue, loss of appetite, and nausea and vomiting.

Cantaloupe Shake

Yield: 1 serving
Preparation time: 10 minutes

1 ½ cups vanilla-flavored
   low-fat yogurt

½ ripe cantaloupe, peeled,
   seeded, and chopped

¼ cup low-fat milk

2 teaspoons lemon juice,
   preferably fresh-squeezed

1 teaspoon vanilla extract

Cantaloupe has more beta-carotene than any other melon. It is usually available throughout the year, with the peak cantaloupe season running from June through August.

1. Put all the ingredients into a blender, and blend until smooth.

NUTRITION INFORMATION (PER SERVING):

Calories: 590   Fat: 6 g   Carbohydrate: 120 g   Protein: 22 g

---

Good for alterations in taste, chewing and swallowing difficulties, dry mouth, fatigue, loss of appetite, nausea and vomiting, and weight gain.

Modification

If experiencing mouth and throat sores, omit the lemon juice. The nutrition information doesn't change.

Carrot Shake

Yield: 1 serving
Preparation time: 10 minutes

1 cup carrot juice

1 cup vanilla-flavored low-fat yogurt

1 medium-sized ripe banana, sliced

1 teaspoon vanilla extract

2 ice cubes

This delicious drink provides a day's dose of beta-carotene at a shot.

1. Put all the ingredients into a blender, and blend until smooth.

NUTRITION INFORMATION (PER SERVING):
Calories: 460   Fat: 5 g   Carbohydrate: 90 g   Protein: 16 g

---

Good for chewing and swallowing difficulties, dry mouth, fatigue, mouth and throat sores, nausea and vomiting, and weight gain.

Cranberry Punch

Yield: 2 servings
Preparation time: 10 minutes

1 ½ cups orange sherbet

1 ½ cups cranberry juice

2 cans (8 ounces each) crushed pineapple, with juice

¾ cup light tofu, drained

This is a thoroughly refreshing beverage for a warm day.

1. Put all the ingredients into a blender, and blend until smooth.

NUTRITION INFORMATION (PER SERVING):
Calories: 495   Fat: 8 g   Carbohydrate: 102 g   Protein: 10 g

---

Good for alterations in taste, chewing and swallowing difficulties, diarrhea, dry mouth, fatigue, loss of appetite, and nausea and vomiting.

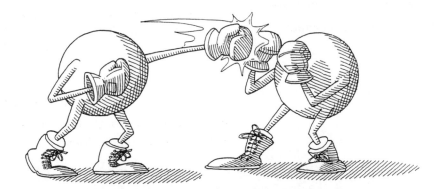

Creamy Berry and Chocolate Shake

Yield: 1 serving
Preparation time: 10 minutes

1 ¼ cups strawberries,
   well-washed fresh or thawed
   frozen

1 ¼ cups low-fat milk

½ cup ricotta cheese

3 tablespoons sugar

2 tablespoons chocolate syrup

1 teaspoon vanilla extract

3 or 4 ice cubes

Strawberries have more vitamin C than any other berry, and half a cup supplies more fiber than a slice of whole wheat bread. Strawberry season is at its peak from April through July.

1. Put all the ingredients into a blender, and blend until smooth.

NUTRITION INFORMATION (PER SERVING):

Calories: 630   Fat: 16 g   Carbohydrate: 100 g   Protein: 26 g

---

Good for chewing and swallowing difficulties, dry mouth,
fatigue, mouth and throat sores, and weight gain.

Fortified Milk

Yield: 4 servings
Preparation time: 5 minutes

1 quart low-fat milk or light
   soymilk

1 cup nonfat dry milk powder or
   soymilk powder

Fortified milk can be used in any recipe that calls for milk. It will add calories and provide an extra boost of protein.

1. Either stir the ingredients together with a spoon, or blend in a blender. Chill.

NUTRITION INFORMATION (PER SERVING):

Calories: 185   Fat: 5 g   Carbohydrate: 21 g   Protein: 14 g

---

Good for every symptom.

Fruit Salad Shake

Yield: 1 serving
Preparation time: 10 minutes

1 can (16 ounces) fruit cocktail,
  with juice

1 cup low-fat milk

½ cup low-fat cottage cheese

If you have extra-ripe fruit that needs to be eaten, use it in this recipe instead of the canned fruit cocktail. Make sure to thoroughly wash all fresh fruit.

1. Put all the ingredients into a blender, and blend until smooth.

NUTRITION INFORMATION (PER SERVING):
Calories: 300   Fat: 7 g   Carbohydrate: 37 g   Protein: 25 g

---

Good for chewing and swallowing difficulties, dry mouth,
fatigue, loss of appetite, mouth and throat sores,
and nausea and vomiting.

Ginger Punch

Yield: 1 serving
Preparation time: 10 minutes

1 cup ginger ale

1 cup unsweetened applesauce

½ cup orange juice

⅓ cup lemon juice, preferably
  fresh-squeezed

This fizzy, tart drink is good for settling the stomach while energizing the body.

1. Stir all the ingredients together until thoroughly mixed, and chill.

NUTRITION INFORMATION (PER SERVING):
Calories: 260   Fat: less than 1 g   Carbohydrate: 66 g   Protein: 1 g

---

Good for alterations in taste, chewing and swallowing difficulties,
diarrhea, dry mouth, fatigue, loss of appetite,
and nausea and vomiting.

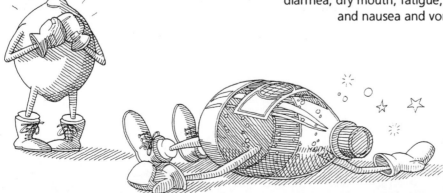

Go Ape Shake

Yield: 2 servings
Preparation time: 10 minutes

2 medium-sized ripe bananas, sliced

1 ½ cups vanilla-flavored low-fat yogurt

1 cup low-fat milk

1 package instant breakfast, any flavor

3 tablespoons honey

Bananas contain less water than most other fruits and, therefore, have a very high carbohydrate content. They also provide loads of potassium, a mineral lost through night sweats, diarrhea, and vomiting.

1. Put all the ingredients into a blender, and blend until smooth.

NUTRITION INFORMATION (PER SERVING):

Calories: 450   Fat: 4 g   Carbohydrate: 88 g   Protein: 16 g

Good for chewing and swallowing difficulties, dry mouth, fatigue, loss of appetite, mouth and throat sores, and weight gain.

Honey Graham Shake

Yield: 1 serving
Preparation time: 10 minutes

1 cup low-fat milk

8 ½-x-2 ½-inch graham crackers, crumbled

2 tablespoons honey

⅛ teaspoon ground cinnamon

Yes, you can put graham crackers in a blender drink! It's an easy way to boost the energy content while adding a mild flavor.

1. Put all the ingredients into a blender, and blend until smooth.

NUTRITION INFORMATION (PER SERVING):

Calories: 390   Fat: 9 g   Carbohydrate: 70 g   Protein: 10 g

Good for chewing and swallowing difficulties, dry mouth, fatigue, loss of appetite, mouth and throat sores, and weight gain.

Modification

If experiencing diarrhea, omit the low-fat milk, and use 1 cup light soymilk or lactose-reduced milk.

MODIFIED NUTRITION INFORMATION:

Calories: 360   Fat: 6 g   Carbohydrate: 73 g   Protein: 6 g

Lemon Blend

Yield: 1 serving
Preparation time: 10 minutes

1 cup lemon-flavored low-fat yogurt

¾ cup low-fat milk

1 medium-sized ripe banana, sliced

1 teaspoon vanilla extract

This drink will give you a refreshing lift as either a snack or a dessert.

1. Put all the ingredients into a blender, and blend until smooth.

NUTRITION INFORMATION (PER SERVING):
Calories: 440   Fat: 7 g   Carbohydrate: 80 g   Protein: 17 g

---

Good for alterations in taste, chewing and swallowing difficulties, dry mouth, loss of appetite, nausea and vomiting, and weight gain.

Mid-Morning Pickup

Yield: 1 serving
Preparation time: 10 minutes

½ cup prune juice

½ cup apple juice

2 tablespoons creamy peanut butter

½ cup plain low-fat yogurt

Prunes, which are dried plums, are known for their naturally sweet taste and laxative effect. But you don't have to eat prunes to get all of their benefits. Prune juice, like the fruit, is a good source of iron, potassium, fiber, and calories.

1. Put all the ingredients into a blender, and blend until smooth.

NUTRITION INFORMATION (PER SERVING):
Calories: 410   Fat: 18 g   Carbohydrates: 52 g   Protein: 15 g

---

Good for chewing and swallowing difficulties, constipation, dry mouth, fatigue, loss of appetite, mouth and throat sores, and weight gain.

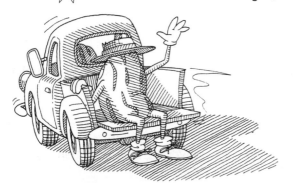

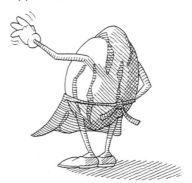

Monster Mango Mash

Yield: 2 servings
Preparation time: 10 minutes

1 ripe, well-washed mango,
  peeled and sliced

1 medium-sized ripe banana,
  sliced

1 cup low-fat milk

1 cup plain low-fat yogurt

2 or 3 ice cubes

Get a blast of beta-carotene, vitamin C, and potassium in this light-tasting, smooth shake.

1. Put all the ingredients into a blender, and blend until smooth.

NUTRITION INFORMATION (PER SERVING):

Calories: 250   Fat: 5 g   Carbohydrate: 45 g   Protein: 11 g

---

Good for chewing and swallowing difficulties, constipation,
dry mouth, fatigue, loss of appetite, mouth and throat sores,
and nausea and vomiting.

Nutty Whip

Yield: 1 serving
Preparation time: 10 minutes

3 tablespoons carob powder*

2 tablespoons nonfat dry milk
  powder

2 tablespoons honey

¼ cup creamy peanut butter

1 large ripe banana, sliced

2 cups low-fat milk

***Carob powder is a chocolate
substitute that has less fat than
chocolate and no caffeine.**

Peanut butter was developed by a St. Louis physician in the 1890s for elderly patients who could not chew peanuts. It is a rich source of protein, B vitamins, phosphorus, magnesium, and iron. Natural peanut butters are your best choice—they are made from peanuts only, with no sugar or hydrogenated oils added.

1. Put all the ingredients into a blender, and blend until smooth.

NUTRITION INFORMATION (PER SERVING):

Calories: 510   Fat: 21 g   Carbohydrate: 68 g   Protein: 18 g

---

Good for chewing and swallowing difficulties, dry mouth, fatigue,
mouth and throat sores, and weight gain.

Peach Smoothie

Yield: 1 serving
Preparation time: 10 minutes

½ cup light tofu, drained

1 cup peach-flavored low-fat yogurt

½ cup peach slices, canned or well-washed fresh

1 or 2 ice cubes

You don't have to peel your fresh peaches before blending (unless you're experiencing diarrhea), but remember to wash them thoroughly.

1. Put all the ingredients into a blender, and blend until smooth.

NUTRITION INFORMATION (PER SERVING):
Calories: 380   Fat: 8 g   Carbohydrate: 60 g   Protein: 21 g

Good for alterations in taste, chewing and swallowing difficulties, dry mouth, fatigue, loss of appetite, mouth and throat sores, nausea and vomiting, and weight gain.

Winter Warmer

Yield: 1 serving
Preparation time: 10 to 15 minutes

1 cup low-fat milk

¼ cup nonfat dry milk powder

1 package chocolate-flavored instant breakfast drink mix

This is a delicious, quick comfort drink that will warm your spirits on the chilliest of days.

1. Place the milk and milk powder in a small saucepan, and heat until the mixture starts to steam—about 5 minutes. Add the instant breakfast mix, and stir. Serve immediately.

NUTRITION INFORMATION (PER SERVING):
Calories: 315   Fat: 6 g   Carbohydrate: 44 g   Protein: 21 g

Good for chewing and swallowing difficulties, dry mouth, fatigue, loss of appetite, and weight gain.

Microwave Cooking

Place the milk and milk powder in a microwave-safe bowl, and microwave on high power for 2 to 3 minutes. Add the instant breakfast mix, and stir. Serve immediately.

Pear Icey

Yield: 1 serving
Preparation time: 10 minutes

1 cup pear halves, canned or
  well-washed and peeled fresh

¼ cup sugar

1 tablespoon lemon juice,
  preferably fresh-squeezed

1 cup crushed ice

This refreshing beverage is best when made with fresh, ripe pears, but canned pears are an acceptable substitute.

1. Put all the ingredients into a blender, and blend until smooth.

NUTRITION INFORMATION (PER SERVING):

Calories: 305   Fat: less than 1 g   Carbohydrate: 81 g   Protein: 1 g

Good for alterations in taste, chewing and swallowing difficulties,
diarrhea, dry mouth, loss of appetite, and nausea and vomiting.

Raspberry Rice Smoothie

Yield: 1 serving
Preparation time: 10 minutes

½ cup cooked brown rice,
  cooled

1 medium-sized ripe banana,
  sliced

1 cup frozen, unsweetened
  raspberries

1 cup plain low-fat yogurt

¼ cup low-fat milk

1 tablespoon honey

Using leftover rice is a great way to boost the carbohydrate content of any smoothie. If the result is too thick, add more liquid to get the consistency you desire. If you don't have leftover rice, see page 213 for rice-cooking instructions.

1. Put all the ingredients into a blender, and blend until smooth.

NUTRITION INFORMATION (PER SERVING):

Calories: 710   Fat: 6 g   Carbohydrate: 150 g   Protein: 19 g

Good for alterations in taste, chewing and swallowing difficulties,
constipation, dry mouth, fatigue, loss of appetite,
mouth and throat sores, nausea and vomiting, and weight gain.

Spicy Squash Smoothie

Yield: 1 serving
Preparation time: 10 minutes

½ cup cooked butternut
  squash, chilled

¼ cup light tofu, drained

1 tablespoon honey

½ cup low-fat milk

⅛ teaspoon ground ginger

⅛ teaspoon pumpkin pie spice

Butternut squash is available all year, and is loaded with beta-carotene.

1. Put all the ingredients into a blender, and blend until smooth.

NUTRITION INFORMATION (PER SERVING):
Calories: 225   Fat: 5 g   Carbohydrate: 36 g   Protein: 14 g

---

Good for alterations in taste, chewing and swallowing difficulties,
dry mouth, fatigue, loss of appetite, mouth and throat sores,
and nausea and vomiting.

Modification

If experiencing diarrhea, omit the low-fat milk, and use $^1\!/_2$ cup light
soymilk or lactose-reduced milk.

MODIFIED NUTRITION INFORMATION:
Calories: 211   Fat: 3 g   Carbohydrate: 38 g   Protein: 12 g

---

Orange Pineapple Delight

Yield: 1 serving
Preparation time: 10 minutes

½ cup orange juice

½ cup pineapple juice

1 medium-sized ripe banana,
  sliced

½ cup light tofu, drained

*Using tofu, a soybean curd, is an easy way to add protein and thickness to
shakes and smoothies.*

1. Put all the ingredients into a blender, and blend until smooth.

NUTRITION INFORMATION (PER SERVING):
Calories: 345   Fat: 5 g   Carbohydrate: 61 g   Protein: 20 g

---

Good for alterations in taste, chewing and swallowing difficulties,
dry mouth, loss of appetite, nausea and vomiting, and weight gain.

Strawberry Delight

Yield: 1 serving
Preparation time: 10 minutes

½ cup strawberries, well-washed fresh or thawed frozen

1 large ripe banana, sliced

1 cup orange juice

1 cup plain low-fat yogurt

2 or 3 ice cubes

Drinking this smoothie is like drinking a sweet-yet-tart candy, but with less sugar and more vitamin C.

1. Put all the ingredients into a blender, and blend until smooth.

NUTRITION INFORMATION (PER SERVING):

Calories: 375   Fat: 5 g   Carbohydrate: 73 g   Protein: 15 g

Good for alterations in taste, chewing and swallowing difficulties, dry mouth, fatigue, loss of appetite, nausea and vomiting, and weight gain.

Modification

If experiencing diarrhea, omit the yogurt, and use 1 cup light soymilk or lactose-reduced milk and ¼ cup light tofu.

MODIFIED NUTRITION INFORMATION:

Calories: 380   Fat: 5 g   Carbohydrate: 74 g   Protein: 16 g

Southern Buttermilk Cooler

Yield: 1 serving
Preparation time: 10 minutes

½ cup dried apricot halves

½ cup pear slices, canned or well-washed and peeled fresh

¾ cup buttermilk (see page 103)

1 medium-sized, ripe banana, sliced

2 or 3 ice cubes

Dried apricots add potassium, iron, and fiber to this tangy-sweet cooler.

1. Put all the ingredients into a blender, and blend until smooth.

NUTRITION INFORMATION (PER SERVING):

Calories: 395   Fat: 3 g   Carbohydrate: 92 g   Protein: 10 g

Good for chewing and swallowing difficulties, constipation, dry mouth, fatigue, loss of appetite, mouth and throat sores, nausea and vomiting, and weight gain.

Sustainable Snacks

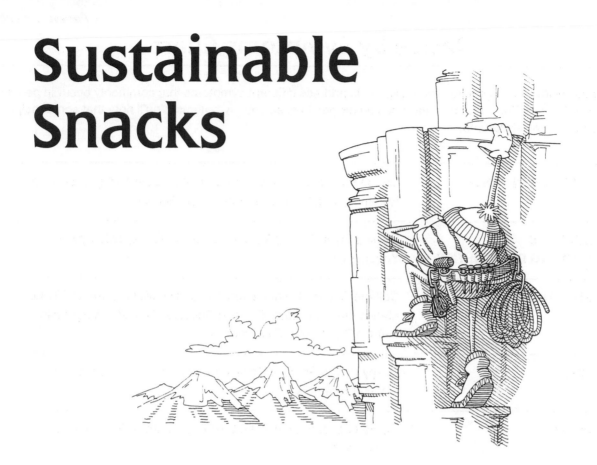

Giving yourself permission to snack between meals may be one of the biggest changes in your routine. But it's the right thing to do! During times of illness, your body requires more nutrients to function at its peak. Simply eating three meals a day will probably not provide you with all the required calories and nutrients. Snacking is a good way to help meet your increased needs.

Keep in mind that the idea is *not* to fill up on simple sugars or foods high in fat. The idea is to eat foods high in carbohydrates and proteins, which will provide you with energy throughout the day. We provide a range of snack recipes—from basic trail mix to several tasty dips to some yummy potato creations—in order to satisfy a variety of cravings.

Make it a practice to prepare snacks ahead of time so that they can be kept on hand for mindless snacking throughout the day. Some recipes, such as Banana Grahams, Cereal Party Mix, and Trail Mix, are portable and can be enjoyed at work or play. Always make sure, however, that you store perishable snacks properly to avoid food-borne illness.

Recipe-by-Symptoms Chart

Different recipes in this section are designed to address different symptoms that commonly occur in people with HIV disease. This chart can help you find recipes to ease your symptoms. You'll note that some recipes address multiple symptoms.

ALTERATIONS IN TASTE	Cereal Party Mix, Crispy Potato Snacks, Deviled Eggs, Low-Fat Hummus, Mediterranean Potato, Tofu Spread
CHEWING AND SWALLOWING DIFFICULTIES	Deviled Eggs, Fruited Tofu, Low-Fat Hummus, Tofu Spread, Yogurt Plus
CONSTIPATION	Cottage Cheese Potato, Crunchy English Muffins, Fruited Tofu, Mediterranean Potato, Spinach Squares, Trail Mix, Vegetable Garden Dip, Yogurt Plus (modified)
DIARRHEA	Crispy Potato Snacks, Deviled Eggs (modified), Fruited Tofu, Low-Fat Hummus
DRY MOUTH	Deviled Eggs, Fruited Tofu, Low-Fat Hummus, Tofu Spread, Yogurt Plus
FATIGUE	Banana Grahams, Cereal Party Mix, Cheesecake Sandwiches, Cottage Cheese Potato, Crunchy English Muffins, Fruited Tofu, Nutty Banana Pops, Quick Cinnamon Spread, Tofu Spread, Trail Mix, Vegetable Garden Dip, Yogurt Plus
LOSS OF APPETITE	Cereal Party Mix, Cheesecake Sandwiches, Cottage Cheese Potato, Crispy Potato Snacks, Crunchy English Muffins, Deviled Eggs, Low-Fat Hummus, Mediterranean Potato, Quick Cinnamon Spread, Tofu Spread, Trail Mix, Yogurt Plus
MOUTH AND THROAT SORES	Cottage Cheese Potato, Deviled Eggs (modified), Fruited Tofu, Low-Fat Hummus, Spinach Squares, Tofu Spread (modified), Yogurt Plus
NAUSEA AND VOMITING	Cereal Party Mix, Cottage Cheese Potato, Crispy Potato Snacks, Deviled Eggs, Low-Fat Hummus, Yogurt Plus

WEIGHT GAIN Banana Grahams, Cereal Party Mix, Cheesecake Sandwiches, Cottage Cheese Potato, Crispy Potato Snacks, Crunchy English Muffins, Fruited Tofu (modified), Mediterranean Potato, Nutty Banana Pops, Quick Cinnamon Spread, Spinach Squares, Tofu Spread, Trail Mix

Banana Grahams

Yield: 1 serving
Preparation time: 5 minutes

2 tablespoons peanut butter

2 4 ½-x-2 ½-inch square
   graham crackers

4 thin slices ripe banana

Prepare these treats ahead of time, and wrap them individually for grab-on-the-go snacks.

1. Spread the peanut butter on one graham cracker. Place the banana slices on top of the peanut butter.

2. Place the other graham cracker on top of the banana slices.

NUTRITION INFORMATION (PER SERVING):

Calories: 310   Fat: 18 g   Carbohydrate: 32 g   Protein: 10 g

---

Good for fatigue and weight gain.

Cereal Party Mix

Yield: 4 servings
Preparation time: 55 minutes

2 tablespoons butter

½ teaspoon seasoned salt

2 teaspoons Worcestershire
   sauce

1 cup crispy rice-square cereal

1 ½ cups crispy wheat-square
   cereal

1 cup thin pretzel sticks

This is a classic recipe that is surprisingly easy to make!

1. Preheat the oven to 250°F.

2. Melt the butter in a large saucepan over medium heat. Stir in the salt and Worcestershire sauce. Add the remaining ingredients, and stir to coat.

3. Pour the mixture into a 9-x-13-inch baking dish. Bake for 45 minutes, stirring every 15 minutes.

4. Spread on a piece of wax paper or a paper towel to cool. Serve immediately, or store in an airtight container for up to 1 month.

NUTRITION INFORMATION (PER 1-CUP SERVING):

Calories: 180   Fat: 6 g   Carbohydrate: 29 g   Protein: 3 g

Good for alterations in taste, fatigue, loss of appetite,
nausea and vomiting, and weight gain.

Cheesecake Sandwiches

Yield: 1 serving
Preparation time: 5 minutes

2 teaspoons low-fat cream
  cheese
2 4 ½-x-2 ½-inch graham
  crackers
1 teaspoon jam

Make these sweet snacks when you have extra time, and freeze for up to 2 weeks.

1. Spread the cream cheese on one graham cracker, and spread the jam on top of the cream cheese.

2. Place the other graham cracker on top of the jam. Serve immediately, or wrap tightly in freezer wrap and freeze.

NUTRITION INFORMATION (PER SANDWICH):
Calories: 118   Fat: 4 g   Carbohydrate: 18 g   Protein: 2 g

Good for fatigue, loss of appetite, and weight gain.

Crunchy English Muffins

Yield: 1 serving
Preparation time: 10 minutes

1 well-washed apple, peeled,
  cored, and sliced crosswise
2 slices cheddar cheese
1 English muffin, split in half
2 tablespoons chopped walnuts

This makes a quick and wholesome meal. A toaster oven is all you need.

1. Place one apple slice and one cheese slice on each half of the English muffin.

2. Place the muffin in a toaster oven or under a broiler until the cheese is bubbly, about 3 minutes. Remove from the oven, and garnish with the walnuts. Serve immediately.

NUTRITION INFORMATION (PER MUFFIN):
Calories: 290   Fat: 12 g   Carbohydrate: 38 g   Protein: 9 g

Good for constipation, fatigue, loss of appetite, and weight gain.

Cottage Cheese Potato

Yield: 1 serving
Preparation time: 50 to 60 minutes

1 large, well-washed baking potato

⅔ cup low-fat cottage cheese

1 tablespoon Italian salad dressing

Baked potatoes are great snacks because of their fatigue-fighting carbohydrates. Adding cottage cheese boosts the protein level, and turns a baked potato into a perfect mini-meal.

1. Preheat the oven to 425°F. Poke holes in the potato, and bake for 45 to 60 minutes, or until the potato is soft throughout.

2. Slice the potato open and fluff up with a fork. Spoon on the cottage cheese first, and then the salad dressing. Serve immediately.

NUTRITION INFORMATION (PER POTATO):

Calories: 425   Fat: 10 g   Carbohydrate: 58 g   Protein: 25 g

---

Good for constipation, fatigue, loss of appetite, mouth and throat sores, nausea and vomiting, and weight gain.

Microwave Cooking

Poke holes in the potato, and microwave on high power for 7 to 10 minutes, or until the potato is soft throughout. Slice the potato open and fluff up with a fork. Spoon on the cottage cheese first, and then the salad dressing. Serve immediately.

Crispy Potato Snacks

Yield: 2 servings
Preparation time: 50 minutes

2 egg whites

Seasonings to taste, such as garlic powder, oregano, or chili powder

2 large, well-washed sweet or white potatoes

This is a high-energy, low-fat alternative to French fries that is easy to digest. The hard part is waiting for these treats to bake and cool before popping them in your mouth!

1. Preheat the oven to 375°F.

2. Place the egg whites and seasonings in a medium-sized mixing bowl, and beat together until smooth.

3. Slice the potatoes into ¼-inch slices. Place the potato slices in the egg white mixture, and coat thoroughly.

4. Spray a cookie sheet with nonstick cooking spray. Place the potato slices on the cookie sheet. Do *not* pour the slices onto the sheet—the egg makes a mess!

5. Bake for approximately 15 to 20 minutes, then flip the potato pieces over and bake for 15 to 20 minutes more, or until the potatoes are crispy. Serve the chips immediately with catsup, salad dressing, low-fat yogurt, salt, cocktail sauce, salsa, vinegar, or soy sauce.

NUTRITION INFORMATION (PER SERVING):

Calories: 350   Fat: less than 1 g   Carbohydrate: 77 g   Protein: 10 g

---

Good for alterations in taste, diarrhea (peel potatoes), loss of appetite, nausea and vomiting, and weight gain.

Fruited Tofu

Yield: 2 servings
Preparation time: 10 minutes

½ pound light tofu, drained (about 1 cup)

1 ripe banana, sliced

½ cup strawberry halves, well-washed fresh or thawed frozen

2 tablespoons honey

This is a refreshing way to benefit from the nutrition of tofu. It's wonderful with graham crackers.

1. Place the tofu, banana, and strawberries in a medium-sized bowl, and mash together with a fork.

2. Stir in the honey. Serve immediately.

NUTRITION INFORMATION (PER SERVING):

Calories: 235   Fat: 4 g   Carbohydrate: 37 g   Protein: 17 g

---

Good for chewing and swallowing difficulties, constipation, diarrhea, dry mouth, fatigue, and mouth and throat sores.

Modification

If weight gain is needed, omit the strawberries, and use ¼ cup raisins.

MODIFIED NUTRITION INFORMATION:

Calories: 285   Fat: 4 g   Carbohydrate: 50 g   Protein: 17 g

---

Mediterranean Potato

Yield: 2 servings
Preparation time: 10 minutes to assemble; 55 to 65 minutes to bake (total)

2 large, well-washed baking potatoes

1 package (10 ounces) frozen chopped spinach, thawed and drained

¼ cup crumbled feta cheese

Seasonings to taste, such as garlic or onion powder, salt, and pepper

The spinach in this recipe will provide you with a large dose of beta-carotene and folate.

1. Preheat the oven to 425°F. Poke holes in the potatoes, and bake for 45 to 60 minutes, or until the potatoes are soft throughout.

2. Slice the potatoes in half lengthwise, and scoop out the flesh with a spoon. Save the shells.

3. Place the potato flesh, spinach, cheese, and seasonings in a medium-sized bowl, and mix thoroughly. Spoon the mixture back into the potato shells.

4. Bake for 10 minutes longer. Serve immediately.

NUTRITION INFORMATION (PER POTATO):

Calories: 345   Fat: 7 g   Carbohydrate: 60 g   Protein: 14 g

---

Good for alterations in taste, constipation, loss of appetite, and weight gain.

Microwave Cooking

Poke holes in the potato, and microwave on high power for 7 to 10 minutes, or until the potatoes are soft throughout. Slice the potatoes in half lengthwise, and scoop out the flesh with a spoon. Save the shells. Place the potato flesh, spinach, cheese, and seasonings in a medium-sized bowl, and mix thoroughly. Spoon the mixture back into the potato shells, and microwave on high power for 1 to 2 minutes. Serve immediately.

Deviled Eggs

Yield: 8 servings
Preparation time: 15 minutes to assemble; 1 hour to chill

8 hard-boiled eggs, shelled

1 cup plain low-fat yogurt

2 tablespoons sweet pickle relish, drained

1 tablespoon prepared mustard, preferably Dijon

¼ teaspoon salt

½ teaspoon white pepper

⅛ teaspoon ground paprika

This high-protein snack can also serve as an appetizer.

1. Slice the eggs in half lengthwise, and remove the yolks. Set the whites aside.

2. Place the yolks in a medium-sized bowl, and mash with a fork. Add the yogurt, relish, mustard, salt, and pepper to the yolk, and mix thoroughly.

3. Spoon about 1 tablespoon of the yolk mixture into each egg white half. Sprinkle with the paprika, then cover and chill for 1 hour before serving. Or, place in an airtight container and store for up to 2 days in the refrigerator.

NUTRITION INFORMATION (PER SERVING):
Calories: 105   Fat: 6 g   Carbohydrate: 4 g   Protein: 8 g

Good for alterations in taste, chewing and swallowing difficulties, dry mouth, loss of appetite, and nausea and vomiting.

Modifications

If experiencing diarrhea, omit the yogurt, and use 1 cup light, drained tofu. Use 12 eggs instead of 8. Set aside 16 of the 24 egg white halves for stuffing. Combine the remaining egg white halves with 4 yolks in a medium-sized bowl, and mash with a fork.

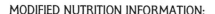

MODIFIED NUTRITION INFORMATION:
Calories: 95   Fat: 4 g   Carbohydrate: 3 g   Protein: 17 g

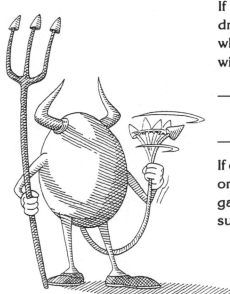

If experiencing mouth and throat sores, omit the relish and mustard, or only use as much as you can tolerate. You may also try onion or garlic powder, or mild herbs such as dill or basil—see what amount suits you. The nutrition information doesn't change.

Low-Fat Hummus

Yield: 4 servings
Preparation time: 10 minutes to
assemble; 1 hour to chill

1 can (15 ounces) garbanzo
   beans, rinsed and drained

2 tablespoons chopped chives

2 cloves garlic, minced

3 tablespoons lemon juice

¼ cup light tofu, drained

2 tablespoons garlic powder

½ teaspoon salt

¼ teaspoon black pepper

½ teaspoon dried dill, or 1
   teaspoon chopped fresh

¼ cup water

We suggest serving this delicious Middle Eastern dish with pita bread.

1. Place all the ingredients in a food processor or blender and purée, adding more water if needed. Pour into a medium-sized bowl.

2. Cover, and chill for at least 1 hour before serving. Serve immediately, or place in an airtight container and store for up to 3 days in the refrigerator.

NUTRITION INFORMATION (PER SERVING):

Calories: 130   Fat: 2 g   Carbohydrate: 20 g   Protein: 7 g

Good for alterations in taste, chewing and swallowing difficulties, diarrhea, dry mouth, loss of appetite, mouth and throat sores, and nausea and vomiting.

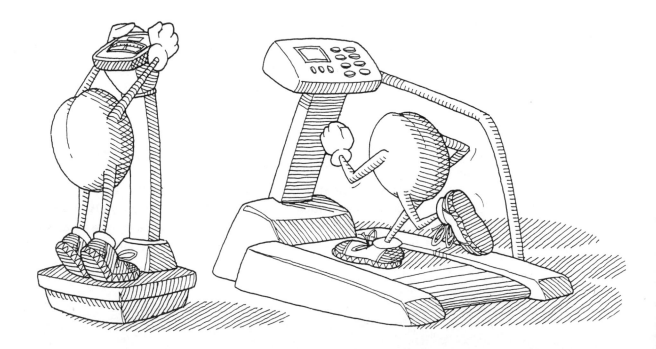

Nutty Banana Pops

Yield: 4 servings
Preparation time: 10 minutes to assemble; 2 hours to freeze

½ cup peanut butter

2 tablespoons low-fat milk

2 ripe bananas

½ cup chopped nuts

A cold glass of milk is the perfect accompaniment for one of these frosty pops. They can be frozen for up to 3 months.

1. Place the peanut butter and milk in small bowl, and mix thoroughly.

2. Cut the bananas in half crosswise, and insert a popsicle stick into each cut end.

3. Spread the peanut butter mixture on the bananas, and then roll the bananas in the chopped nuts.

4. Place the bananas on a cookie sheet covered with waxed paper, and freeze until firm—about 2 hours. When frozen, place in an airtight container.

NUTRITION INFORMATION (PER POP):

Calories: 350   Fat: 26 g   Carbohydrate: 24 g   Protein: 13 g

Good for fatigue and weight gain.

Quick Cinnamon Spread

Yield: 8 servings
Preparation time: 5 minutes

½ cup butter, softened

½ cup sugar

1 teaspoon ground nutmeg

2 teaspoons ground cinnamon

Don't wait until you're overcome with hunger to prepare this quick-and-easy spread. Keep it on hand to use on muffins, pancakes, waffles, and toast.

1. Place all the ingredients in a small bowl, and beat together until fluffy. Serve immediately, or place in an airtight container and store for up to 2 weeks in the refrigerator.

NUTRITION INFORMATION (PER SERVING):

Calories: 140   Fat: 7 g   Carbohydrate: 18 g   Protein: 3 g

Good for fatigue, loss of appetite, and weight gain.

Spinach Squares

Yield: 4 servings
Preparation time: 40 minutes

These squares make delicious appetizers. They also make hearty snacks when served with crackers, French bread, or baguettes.

2 packages (10 ounces each) frozen chopped spinach, thawed and drained

½ cup chopped onion

1 cup low-fat cottage cheese

½ cup shredded mozzarella cheese

2 eggs

1. Preheat the oven to 350°F.

2. Spray a 9-x-9-inch baking dish with nonstick cooking spray. Press the spinach into the dish, and sprinkle with the onions.

3. Place the cottage cheese, ¼ cup of the mozzarella cheese, and the eggs in a medium-sized bowl, and mix thoroughly. Pour the cheese mixture over the spinach, and sprinkle with the remaining ¼ cup of mozzarella cheese.

4. Bake for 20 minutes, or until firm. Cut into 4 squares, and serve immediately.

NUTRITION INFORMATION (PER SQUARE):
Calories: 215   Fat: 11 g   Carbohydrate: 10 g   Protein: 21 g

---

Good for constipation, mouth and throat sores, and weight gain.

Trail Mix

Yield: 8 servings
Preparation time: 5 minutes

This is another on-the-go, nutrient-dense treat. This recipe can be altered to include your favorite snack foods, such as coconut flakes, dates, any type of nuts, seeds, cereals, and various dried fruits.

1 cup raisins

1 cup roasted peanuts

1 cup chocolate chips

1 cup banana chips

1. Place all the ingredients in an airtight container, and mix thoroughly. Serve immediately, or store for up to 2 weeks in the refrigerator.

NUTRITION INFORMATION (PER SERVING):
Calories: 305   Fat: 18 g   Carbohydrate: 36 g   Protein: 6 g

---

Good for constipation, fatigue, loss of appetite, and weight gain.

Tofu Spread

Yield: 8 servings
Preparation time: 10 minutes

1 ⅓ cups tofu, drained

½ cup creamy peanut butter

2 ripe bananas, sliced

2 tablespoons lemon juice,
    preferably fresh-squeezed

2 tablespoons honey

Serve this spread on a hearty piece of whole grain bread. Or, top it with nuts, raisins, or sliced bananas, and eat it with a spoon. It's also good when frozen until just firm.

1. Place all the ingredients in a blender, and purée until smooth. Serve immediately, or place in an airtight container and store for up to 3 days in the refrigerator.

NUTRITION INFORMATION (PER SERVING):
Calories: 175   Fat: 10 g   Carbohydrate: 16 g   Protein: 10 g

Good for alterations in taste, chewing and swallowing difficulties, dry mouth, fatigue, loss of appetite, and weight gain.

Modification

If experiencing mouth and throat sores, omit the lemon juice. The nutrition information doesn't change.

Vegetable Garden Dip

Yield: 2 servings
Preparation time: 5 minutes

1 cup plain low-fat yogurt

¼ cup grated Parmesan cheese

1 package dry soup mix

We suggest serving this refreshing dip with 1½ cups each of well-washed, cut-up broccoli and carrots. Or try it on your favorite raw veggie.

1. Place all the ingredients in a medium-sized bowl, and beat until well blended. Serve immediately, or place in an airtight container and store for up to 3 days in the refrigerator.

NUTRITION INFORMATION (PER SERVING):
Calories: 200   Fat: 6 g   Carbohydrate: 26 g   Protein: 14 g

Good for constipation and fatigue.

Yogurt Plus

Yield: 2 servings
Preparation time: 5 minutes to assemble; 2 hours to chill

1 cup plain low-fat yogurt

½ cup unsweetened applesauce

½ teaspoon ground cinnamon

2 tablespoons wheat bran

This recipe calls for cinnamon to add flavor, and for bran to add fiber and texture. But feel free to try any or all of your favorite toppings—nutmeg, dried fruit, granola, or puréed fruit.

1. Place all the ingredients in a medium-sized bowl, and mix thoroughly. Serve immediately.

NUTRITION INFORMATION (PER SERVING):

Calories: 110   Fat: 2 g   Carbohydrate: 17 g   Protein: 7 g

Good for chewing and swallowing difficulties, dry mouth,
fatigue, loss of appetite, mouth and throat sores,
and nausea and vomiting.

Modification

If experiencing constipation, omit the applesauce, and use $\frac{1}{4}$ cup raisins and 4 dried, chopped figs.

MODIFIED NUTRITION INFORMATION:

Calories: 230   Fat: 3 g   Carbohydrate: 49 g   Protein: 9 g

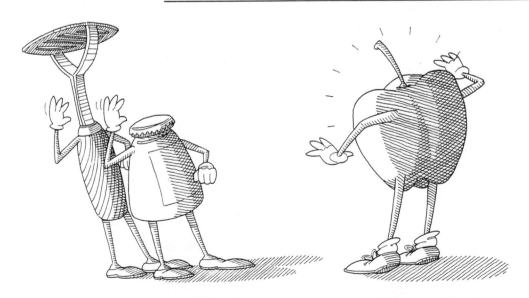

The Salad Bowl

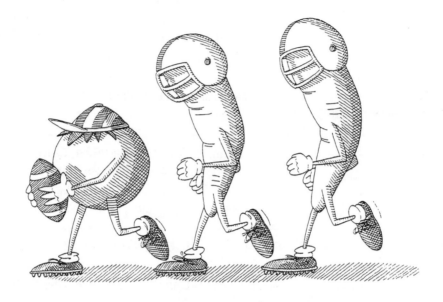

S alad is far more than a wedge of iceberg lettuce and a slice of tomato.
Salads come in all colors and sizes, and can be served as meals in themselves, as accompaniments to a main meal, or as snacks. You can create your own nutrient-dense masterpieces that suit your taste and tolerances by adding leftovers from the refrigerator.

Use dark green lettuces for salads because they contain more nutrients, such as iron, calcium, folate, and beta-carotene, than do iceberg types. Boost the calories and protein value by topping salads with your favorite nuts, cubed or grated cheese, low-fat cottage cheese, low-fat yogurt, diced meats, beans, corn, or peas.

Salads can be great meals for those nights when it's hot and uncomfortable, or when you're just too busy or tired to spend a lot of time in the kitchen. To help speed things along when preparing meals, chop fruits and vegetables ahead of time, and store them in the refrigerator. Remember to thoroughly wash all fruits and vegetables before using them. We recommend not storing salads made with greens for very long—they tend to get soggy, and don't keep very well. Salads made with potatoes, grains, or pasta can generally be stored for about a week.

Recipe-by-Symptoms Chart

Different recipes in this section are designed to address different symptoms that commonly occur in people with HIV disease. This chart can help you find recipes to ease your symptoms. You'll note that some recipes address multiple symptoms.

ALTERATIONS IN TASTE	Artichoke and Tuna, Carrot, Couscous Shrimp, Four-Bean, Fruit and Honey Spinach, Garbanzo and Mushroom, Hearty Cole Slaw, Herb Potato, Poppy Seed Fruit, Tropical Fruit, Vegetarian Taco
CHEWING AND SWALLOWING DIFFICULTIES	Artichoke and Tuna (modified)
CONSTIPATION	Apple-Banana, Carrot, Chilled Rice, Corn and Pea, Couscous Shrimp (modified), Four-Bean, Fruit and Honey Spinach, Garbanzo and Mushroom, Hearty Cole Slaw, Parmesan Pasta (modified), Poppy Seed Fruit, Tropical Fruit, Vegetarian Taco
DIARRHEA	Carrot (modified), Chilled Rice (modified), Herb Potato (modified)
DRY MOUTH	Apple-Banana, Carrot, Chilled Rice, Hearty Cole Slaw, Herb Potato, Tropical Fruit
FATIGUE	Apple-Banana, Artichoke and Tuna, Chilled Rice, Corn and Pea, Couscous Shrimp, Four-Bean, Parmesan Pasta (modified), Vegetarian Taco
LOSS OF APPETITE	Carrot, Chilled Rice, Corn and Pea, Herb Potato, Poppy Seed Fruit, Tropical Fruit
MOUTH AND THROAT SORES	Herb Potato (modified)
NAUSEA AND VOMITING	Carrot, Chilled Rice, Corn and Pea, Fruit and Honey Spinach (modified), Herb Potato, Poppy Seed Fruit, Tropical Fruit
WEIGHT GAIN	Apple-Banana, Artichoke and Tuna, Chilled Rice, Couscous Shrimp, Hearty Cole Slaw, Parmesan Pasta, Vegetarian Taco

Apple-Banana Salad

Yield: 4 servings
Preparation time: 10 minutes

4 well-washed sweet apples,
  cored and cut into bite-sized
  pieces

2 ripe bananas, sliced

½ cup chopped roasted
  peanuts

1 cup plain or vanilla-flavored
  low-fat yogurt

Apples are a good source of fiber. Bananas are a good source of carbohydrates and potassium.

1. Place the apples and bananas in a medium-sized bowl, and mix thoroughly. Add the nuts and yogurt, and toss. Serve immediately, or chill for 1 hour. Leftovers can be placed in an airtight container and stored for up to 3 days in the refrigerator.

NUTRITION INFORMATION (PER SERVING):

Calories: 275   Fat: 11 g   Carbohydrate: 42 g   Protein: 8 g

---

Good for constipation, dry mouth, fatigue, and weight gain.

Corn and Pea Salad

Yield: 2 servings
Preparation time: 10 minutes to
assemble; 1 hour to chill

1 cup peas, thawed frozen or
  canned, drained

1 cup corn kernels, thawed
  frozen or canned, drained

1 ½ cups low-fat cottage
  cheese

1 tablespoon chopped
  well-washed green bell
  pepper

1 tablespoon chopped
  well-washed parsley

1 teaspoon salt

Peas and corn are both good sources of fiber, and they complement each other very well in this colorful salad.

1. Place all the ingredients in a medium-sized bowl, and toss. Chill for about 1 hour. Serve immediately.

NUTRITION INFORMATION (PER SERVING):

Calories: 255   Fat: 4 g   Carbohydrate: 29 g   Protein: 29 g

---

Good for constipation, fatigue, loss of appetite,
and nausea and vomiting.

Artichoke and Tuna Salad

Yield: 2 servings
Preparation time: 15 minutes

3 tablespoons olive oil

1 tablespoon lemon juice,
    preferably fresh-squeezed

1 can (7 ounces) water-packed
    tuna, drained

6 canned artichoke hearts,
    chopped

1 large well-washed tomato, cut
    into thin wedges

2 teaspoons dried dill, or 1
    tablespoon chopped fresh

½ teaspoon salt

1 teaspoon black pepper

3 or 4 well-washed lettuce
    leaves

Eat this tuna treat as is, or use it to either fill a pita pocket or spread on crackers. You can also use it as a dip for vegetables. Artichokes are a rich source of vitamin C and fiber.

1. Place the olive oil and lemon juice in a medium-sized bowl, and mix thoroughly. Add the rest of the ingredients. Mix well.

2. Arrange the lettuce on a serving platter, and place the salad on top. Serve immediately.

NUTRITION INFORMATION (PER SERVING):

Calories: 390   Fat: 22 g   Carbohydrate: 18 g   Protein: 34 g

---

Good for alterations in taste, fatigue, and weight gain.

Modification

If experiencing chewing and swallowing difficulties, omit the tomato, and chop the artichoke hearts finely.

MODIFIED NUTRITION INFORMATION:

Calories: 380   Fat: 22 g   Carbohydrate: 16 g   Protein: 34 g

---

Four-Bean Salad

Yield: 8 servings
Preparation time: 20 minutes to assemble; 2 hours to chill

1 cup canned garbanzo beans, rinsed and drained

1 cup canned kidney beans, rinsed and drained

1 can (16 ounces) green beans, rinsed and drained

1 can (16 ounces) wax beans, rinsed and drained

½ cup chopped onion

½ cup minced well-washed green bell pepper

½ cup vegetable oil

½ cup vinegar

½ cup sugar

1 teaspoon salt

½ teaspoon black pepper

¼ teaspoon prepared mustard

This is our version of an all-time favorite.

1. Remove any loose skins from the garbanzo beans.

2. Place all the beans in a large bowl, and add the onion and green pepper. Mix thoroughly.

3. Make the dressing by placing the remaining ingredients in a medium-sized bowl, and mixing thoroughly. Make sure that the sugar is completely dissolved.

4. Pour the dressing over the beans, and chill, tossing occasionally, for 2 hours. Serve immediately.

NUTRITION INFORMATION (PER SERVING):

Calories: 215   Fat: 14 g   Carbohydrate: 19 g   Protein: 5 g

---

Good for alterations in taste, constipation, and fatigue.

Chilled Rice Salad

Yield: 4 servings
Preparation time: 5 minutes to assemble; 1 hour to chill

1 cup brown or white rice, cooked and drained (measure before cooking)

1 jar (6 ounces) marinated artichoke hearts, chopped (reserve marinade)

1 can (7 ounces) sliced water chestnuts

You can use leftover cooked rice in this simple salad, or you can cook the rice fresh, following the directions on page 213.

1. Place all the ingredients, including the artichoke marinade, in a large bowl, and mix thoroughly. Chill for about 1 hour before serving. Leftovers can be placed in an airtight container and stored for up to 1 week in the refrigerator.

NUTRITION INFORMATION (PER SERVING):
Calories: 280   Fat: 7 g   Carbohydrate: 50 g   Protein: 5 g

Good for constipation (use brown rice), dry mouth, fatigue, loss of appetite, nausea and vomiting, and weight gain.

Modification

If experiencing diarrhea, use white rice. Omit the water chestnuts, and use 1 can (7 ounces) of sliced mushrooms, drained. The nutrition information doesn't change.

Carrot Salad

Yield: 4 servings
Preparation time: 10 minutes to assemble; 1 hour to chill

2 cups grated well-washed carrot (3 to 5 carrots)

½ cup plain low-fat yogurt

½ cup raisins

3 teaspoons honey

½ cup canned pineapple chunks, drained

Carrots are a great source of beta-carotene, and this is a delicious way to serve them.

1. Place all the ingredients in a medium-sized bowl, and toss. Chill for 1 hour before serving. Leftovers can be placed in an airtight container and stored for up to 1 week in the refrigerator.

NUTRITION INFORMATION (PER SERVING):
Calories: 130   Fat: 1 g   Carbohydrate: 31 g   Protein: 3 g

Good for alterations in taste, constipation, dry mouth, loss of appetite, and nausea and vomiting.

Modification

If experiencing diarrhea, omit the raisins and yogurt. Use 1 peeled, cored, and chopped apple, and $\frac{1}{2}$ cup soft light tofu.

MODIFIED NUTRITION INFORMATION:

Calories: 80   Fat: 2 g   Carbohydrate: 15 g   Protein: 3 g

Couscous Shrimp Salad

Yield: 4 servings
Preparation time: 25 minutes to assemble; 1 hour to chill

2 cups water

1 cup uncooked couscous*

1 ½ cups chopped well-washed tomato

½ cup finely chopped well-washed parsley

2 cans (4 ¼ ounces each) shrimp, drained

⅓ cup lemon juice, preferably fresh-squeezed

3 tablespoons olive oil

1 teaspoon black pepper

½ teaspoon salt

*Couscous is a form of pasta from the Middle East that looks like large grains of sand.

Using canned shrimp makes this salad quick and easy to prepare.

1. Bring the water to a boil in a medium-sized saucepan over high heat. Stir in the couscous.

2. Cover, remove from the heat, and let stand for 5 minutes. Fluff with a fork, and cool for 10 minutes.

3. Add the tomatoes, parsley, and shrimp, and toss gently.

4. Place the lemon juice, olive oil, pepper, and salt in a small bowl, and mix thoroughly. Add to the couscous mixture.

5. Transfer the mixture to a serving bowl, and chill—about 1 hour. Serve immediately.

NUTRITION INFORMATION (PER SERVING):

Calories: 365   Fat: 12 g   Carbohydrate: 42 g   Protein: 21 g

---

Good for alterations in taste, fatigue, and weight gain.

Modification

If experiencing constipation, use 1 cup whole wheat couscous. The nutrition information doesn't change.

Fruit and Honey Spinach Salad

Yield: 4 servings
Preparation time: 15 minutes

1 bunch well-washed spinach leaves, drained

2 cups melon balls or cubes (1 small melon)

1 ½ cups halved strawberries, well-washed fresh or thawed frozen

2 tablespoons raspberry jam

2 tablespoons raspberry white wine vinegar

1 tablespoon honey

1 tablespoon olive oil

¼ cup chopped macadamia nuts

This sweet-yet-tart salad is a delicious way to get your vitamins.

1. Place the spinach, melon, and strawberries in a large bowl, and gently toss.

2. Place the jam, vinegar, honey, and oil in a smaller bowl, and mix thoroughly. Add the jam mixture to the spinach mixture, folding it in gently. Sprinkle the nuts on top. Serve immediately.

NUTRITION INFORMATION (PER SERVING):

Calories: 240   Fat: 14 g   Carbohydrate: 28 g   Protein: 5 g

---

Good for alterations in taste and constipation.

Modification

If experiencing nausea and vomiting, omit the nuts, and use ¼ cup cubed firm tofu. Reduce the oil to 2 teaspoons.

MODIFIED NUTRITION INFORMATION:

Calories: 160   Fat: 5 g   Carbohydrate: 27 g   Protein: 7 g

Garbanzo and Mushroom Salad

Yield: 4 servings
Preparation time: 30 minutes to assemble; 1 hour to chill

¾ cup garbanzo beans, cooked fresh or canned, rinsed and drained

1 cup sliced well-washed mushrooms

¼ cup sliced well-washed celery, cut diagonally

¼ cup chopped well-washed red bell pepper

2 tablespoons chopped onion

2 tablespoons chopped well-washed parsley

3 tablespoons olive oil

1 ½ tablespoons red wine vinegar

1 teaspoon garlic powder

1 teaspoon soy sauce

1 teaspoon salt

1 teaspoon black pepper

½ teaspoon cayenne pepper

If you don't have garbanzo beans, try black-eyed peas, or kidney, black, or pinto beans in this salad. If you are cooking the garbanzo beans from scratch, see page 212 for cooking instructions.

1. Place the garbanzo beans, mushrooms, celery, bell pepper, onion, and parsley in a large bowl, and toss.

2. Make the dressing by placing the remaining ingredients in a small bowl, and beating with a wire whisk until smooth.

3. Add the dressing to the garbanzo bean mixture, and mix thoroughly. Chill for about 1 hour. Serve immediately, or place in an airtight container and store for up to 1 week in the refrigerator.

Good for alterations in taste and constipation.

NUTRITION INFORMATION (PER SERVING):			
Calories: 155	Fat: 11 g	Carbohydrate: 11 g	Protein: 3 g

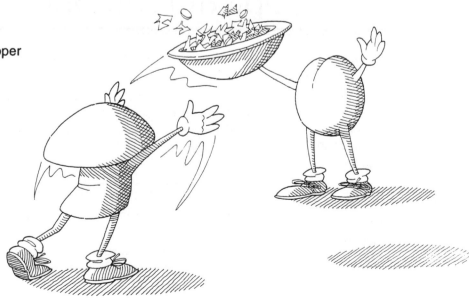

Hearty Cole Slaw

Yield: 4 servings
Preparation time: 20 minutes to assemble; 1 hour to chill

2 cups shredded well-washed cabbage (½ small head)

1 well-washed apple, cored and grated

½ cup grated well-washed carrot

½ cup chopped pecans

½ cup sunflower seeds

1 cup plain low-fat yogurt

2 tablespoons honey

2 tablespoons apple cider vinegar

1 teaspoon salt

Use both red and green cabbages for a more colorful salad. Cabbage is rich in vitamin C.

1. Place the cabbage, apple, carrot, pecans, and sunflower seeds in a large bowl, and mix thoroughly.

2. Stir in the remaining ingredients, and chill for about 1 hour. Serve immediately, or place in an airtight container and store for up to 1 week in the refrigerator.

NUTRITION INFORMATION (PER SERVING):
Calories: 290   Fat: 18 g   Carbohydrate: 28 g   Protein: 8 g

---

Good for alterations in taste, constipation, dry mouth,
and weight gain.

Tropical Fruit Salad

Yield: 4 servings
Preparation time: 15 minutes to assemble; 1 hour to chill

2 cups fresh or canned pineapple chunks, drained

2 ripe bananas, sliced

2 large oranges, peeled and sectioned, or 1 can mandarin oranges, drained

3 tablespoons coconut flakes

2 cups plain low-fat yogurt

This salad is loaded with vitamin C. Try adding raisins or nuts, if you like.

1. Place the pineapple, bananas, and oranges in a large bowl, and gently toss. Stir in the coconut flakes, and chill for about 1 hour. Serve immediately, or place in an airtight container and store for up to 1 week in the refrigerator.

NUTRITION INFORMATION (PER SERVING):
Calories: 230   Fat: 5 g   Carbohydrate: 42 g   Protein: 8 g

Good for alterations in taste, constipation, dry mouth,
loss of appetite, and nausea and vomiting.

Parmesan Pasta Salad

Yield: 4 servings
Preparation time: 10 minutes to assemble; 1 hour to chill

8 ounces pasta, cooked, drained, and cooled (measure before cooking)

2 cups broccoli florets, steamed and cooled

2 tablespoons olive oil

½ cup grated Parmesan cheese

2 well-washed large tomatoes, chopped

This salad works best with the shorter, chewier types of pasta, such as ditali or short fusilli. If you're not sure how to steam the broccoli, see page 178.

1. Place the pasta and broccoli in a large bowl, and mix thoroughly. Add the olive oil, cheese, and tomatoes, and mix thoroughly. Chill for about 1 hour. Serve immediately, or place in an airtight container and store for up to 1 week in the refrigerator.

NUTRITION INFORMATION (PER SERVING):

Calories: 410   Fat: 12 g   Carbohydrate: 59 g   Protein: 18 g

---

Good for weight gain.

Modifications

If experiencing fatigue, omit the fresh broccoli, and use 1 package (10 ounces) frozen broccoli, thawed and drained. The nutrition information doesn't change.

If experiencing constipation, use 8 ounces whole wheat pasta. The nutrition information doesn't change.

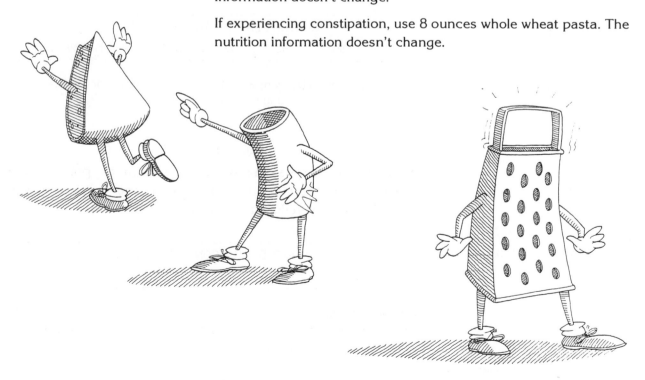

Herb Potato Salad

Yield: 6 servings
Preparation time: 45 minutes to assemble; 2 hours to chill

2 ½ pounds well-washed small, round red potatoes

½ cup well-washed basil leaves

½ cup skim buttermilk (see page 103)

¼ cup plain low-fat yogurt

1 teaspoon salt

1 teaspoon black pepper

¾ cup chopped well-washed scallions

Make a double batch of this salad to snack on throughout the week.

1. Place the potatoes in a large pot. Cover with water, and then cover the pot. Put over high heat, and bring to a boil. Reduce the heat to medium, and simmer the potatoes for 25 minutes until tender, keeping the pot partially covered.

2. While the potatoes are cooking, place the basil, buttermilk, and yogurt in a blender, and blend until smooth. Also, you can hand-chop the basil until fine, and then use a spoon to mix it with the buttermilk and yogurt. Add the salt and pepper to the basil-yogurt mixture, and mix thoroughly.

3. After the potatoes are cooked, drain them, and cool them in cold running water for about 5 minutes. Then cut each potato into eighths, placing the pieces in a large bowl.

4. Add the scallions and the basil-yogurt mixture, and toss until the potato pieces are coated. Cover the bowl, and chill for about 2 hours. Serve immediately, or place in an airtight container and store for up to 1 week in the refrigerator.

NUTRITION INFORMATION (PER SERVING):
Calories: 185   Fat: 1 g   Carbohydrate: 41 g   Protein: 5 g

Good for alterations in taste, dry mouth, loss of appetite,
and nausea and vomiting.

Modifications

If experiencing diarrhea, remove the skins from the potatoes after cooking. Omit the buttermilk and yogurt, and use ½ cup light soymilk or lactose-reduced milk and ¼ cup light tofu.

MODIFIED NUTRITION INFORMATION:
Calories: 155   Fat: 1 g   Carbohydrate: 32 g   Protein: 6 g

If experiencing mouth and throat sores, omit the onions, salt, and pepper as tolerated, and use 1 tablespoon of onion powder. The nutrition information doesn't change.

Poppy Seed Fruit Salad

Yield: 10 servings
Preparation time: 40 minutes to assemble; 1 hour to chill

4 cups halved strawberries, well-washed fresh or thawed frozen

3 cups honeydew melon balls or cubes (1 medium-sized melon)

1 ½ cups well-washed red grapes

1 ½ cups well-washed green grapes

4 well-washed medium-sized peaches, peeled and sliced

2 large ripe bananas, sliced

DRESSING

½ cup sugar

1 teaspoon salt

1 teaspoon dried mustard

¼ cup raspberry vinegar

¼ cup canola oil

1 teaspoon poppy seeds

Preparing the fresh fruit can be time consuming. There are frozen fruit mixtures available that can save you time and energy.

1. Place the strawberries, melon, grapes, and peaches in a large bowl, and toss gently.

2. Place the dressing ingredients in a small bowl, and mix thoroughly. Pour over the fruit, and toss until the fruit is coated. Chill for about 1 hour. Add the bananas just before serving.

NUTRITION INFORMATION (PER SERVING):

Calories: 250   Fat: 8 g   Carbohydrate: 49 g   Protein: 2 g

Good for alterations in taste, constipation, loss of appetite, and nausea and vomiting.

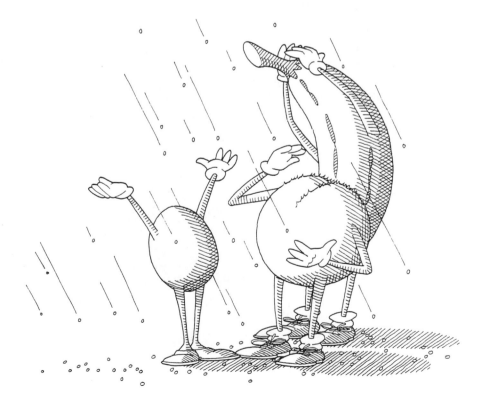

Vegetarian Taco Salad

Yield: 4 servings
Preparation time: 20 minutes

1 tablespoon canola oil

¼ cup chopped onion

¼ cup chopped well-washed green bell pepper

½ teaspoon chili powder

1 can (15 ounces) vegetarian refried beans

4 ounces tortilla chips (about 40 chips)

1 head well-washed lettuce, drained and shredded

1 large well-washed tomato, chopped

1 cup chopped black olives

½ cup prepared salsa

Alter the spices in this zippy salad to suit your tastes and tolerances.

1. Place the oil in a large frying pan over medium heat. Add the onion, green pepper, and chili powder, and sauté until the onion is tender, about 3 minutes. Add the refried beans, and heat through, about 2 minutes.

2. Spread the chips evenly among four plates, and place the lettuce on top of the chips, again dividing evenly.

3. Spoon the bean mixture onto the lettuce, and add the tomatoes and olives. Serve immediately, with the salsa on the side.

NUTRITION INFORMATION (PER SERVING):

Calories: 345   Fat: 17 g   Carbohydrate: 43 g   Protein: 11 g

---

Good for alterations in taste, constipation, fatigue, and weight gain.

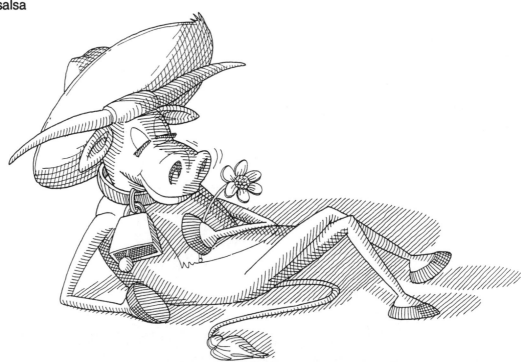

Soup's On

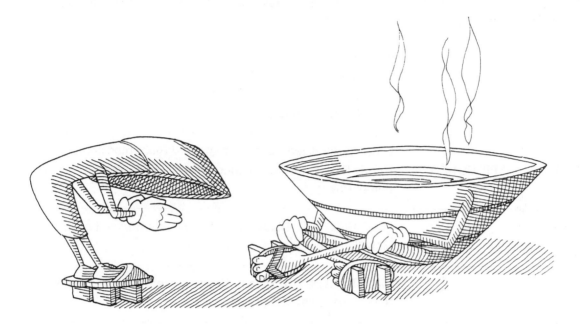

Soups are among the most versatile of foods. They can serve as an appetizer before the entrée, or, when sufficiently hearty, can be a meal in themselves. And, of course, soup makes a nourishing snack.

Not all soups are for cold winter days. One, Potato-Zucchini, can be served chilled— a refreshing summer alternative. Others are so stew-like that you may prefer a fork to the traditional spoon.

Soup is good at any time of the day. One of the benefits of many soup recipes is that you can prepare them ahead of time in bulk, and freeze the soup in individual portions for later use. In fact, the taste of many soups improve the longer the flavors are allowed to blend.

But leftover soup must be cooled properly. Do not let it sit in the pot on the stove to cool. Bacteria will grow, and you will increase your risk of food-borne illness. Transfer portions to shallow bowls, cover, and cool in the refrigerator. Leftover soup that is stored in the refrigerator should be consumed within two to three days. Frozen soup will last up to three months.

Recipe-by-Symptoms Chart

Different recipes in this section are designed to address different symptoms that commonly occur in people with HIV disease. This chart can help you find recipes to ease your symptoms. You'll note that some recipes address multiple symptoms.

ALTERATIONS IN TASTE	Black Bean Chili, Black-Eyed Pea, Easy Tomato and Rice, Hearty Barley, Lentil, McMillan's Minestrone, Potato-Zucchini, Sweet Potato, Turkey Chili
CHEWING AND SWALLOWING DIFFICULTIES	Chicken (modified), Easy Tomato and Rice (modified), Hearty Barley, Instant Mashed Potato, Lentil, Potato-Zucchini, Sweet Potato
CONSTIPATION	Black Bean Chili, Black-Eyed Pea, Hearty Barley, Lentil, McMillan's Minestrone, Turkey Chili
DIARRHEA	Black-Eyed Pea (modified), Chicken, Hearty Barley, Lentil (modified), Sweet Potato (modified)
DRY MOUTH	All
FATIGUE	Black Bean Chili, Black-Eyed Pea, Easy Tomato and Rice, Hearty Barley, Instant Mashed Potato, Lentil, McMillan's Minestrone, Potato-Zucchini, Turkey Chili
LOSS OF APPETITE	Black Bean Chili, Black-Eyed Pea, Chicken, Easy Tomato and Rice, Hearty Barley, Lentil, McMillan's Minestrone, Turkey Chili
MOUTH AND THROAT SORES	Chicken, Instant Mashed Potato, Potato-Zucchini
NAUSEA AND VOMITING	Black-Eyed Pea, Chicken, Easy Tomato and Rice, Hearty Barley, Lentil, Potato-Zucchini, Sweet Potato
WEIGHT GAIN	Black Bean Chili, Instant Mashed Potato, Potato-Zucchini, Sweet Potato, Turkey Chili

Of Stocks and Soups

Stock, or broth, is the basis of most soups. Stock is made by boiling a flavoring agent, such as chicken, beef, or vegetables, in water. There are a number of commercial stocks, in a number of forms: cans, packets of powder, compressed-powder cubes. Try different forms and brands until you find something you like. There are also a number of low-sodium stocks on the market. You may want to try one if you've been told to cut down on your salt intake. If you want to make your own stock—a good rainy-day project—you can use one of these recipes.

Vegetable Stock

Yield: 8 cups
Preparation time: 1 hour

1 teaspoon canola oil

1 medium-sized whole onion, skin removed

1 large clove garlic, halved

1 small, well-washed carrot, peeled and halved

1 small, well-washed celery stalk

2 medium-sized, well-washed potatoes, peeled and diced

8 cups water

6 peppercorns

½ teaspoon celery seeds

This nourishing stock can be used in any vegetable- or beef-based soup recipe.

1. Place the oil in a large pot over medium-high heat. Add the onion, and sauté for 2 minutes. Add the garlic, and sauté for another minute.

2. Add the remaining ingredients. Reduce the heat to medium, and simmer, uncovered, for 1 hour.

3. Use a slotted spoon to remove the vegetables, which should be discarded.

Chicken Stock

Yield: 8 cups
Preparation time: 2 hours to cook;
6 hours to chill

1 3-pound chicken

Water

1 large, well-washed carrot, peeled

1 small whole onion, skin removed

1 large, well-washed celery stalk

½ teaspoon black pepper

½ teaspoon celery seeds

This stock takes a while to make, but it's delicious. Use it in any vegetable- or chicken-based soup recipe.

1. Place the chicken in a large pot over high heat, and completely cover with water. Bring to a boil, reduce the heat to low, and skim any foam off the top.

2. Add the remaining ingredients, cover the pot, and simmer for 1½ hours, or until the chicken is tender.

3. Remove the chicken, which can be used in any recipe that calls for boiled chicken. Use a slotted spoon to remove the vegetables, which should be discarded.

4. Cover the pot, and refrigerate for 6 hours.

5. Skim the fat off the top of the cooled stock.

Black-Eyed Pea Soup

Yield: 4 servings
Preparation time: 3 hours (after soaking the peas overnight)

2 cups dried black-eyed peas (about 1 pound)

3 quarts water, divided

2 medium-sized, well-washed potatoes, diced

3 well-washed celery stalks, sliced

2 well-washed carrots, peeled and sliced

1 medium-sized onion, chopped

1 can (15 ounces) tomato sauce

3 tablespoons soy sauce

2 teaspoons black pepper

1 teaspoon dried basil

1 teaspoon dried dill

1 teaspoon salt

This is a very comforting soup with a mild flavor.

1. Rinse the black-eyed peas well, then place in a large pot and cover with 6 cups (1 ½ quarts) of the water. Soak overnight.

2. Drain the peas, return to the pot, and cover with the remaining 6 cups of water. Add the rest of the ingredients. Place the pot over high heat, and bring to a boil. Boil for 5 minutes.

3. Reduce the heat to medium-low. Simmer for 1 to 2 hours, or until the peas are tender. Stir occasionally. For a thicker soup, mash the peas and potatoes against the sides of the pot while stirring. Serve hot.

NUTRITION INFORMATION (PER SERVING):

Calories: 270   Fat: 1 g   Carbohydrate: 61 g   Protein: 8 g

Good for alterations in taste, constipation, dry mouth, loss of appetite, and nausea and vomiting. If fatigued, make a double batch and freeze for up to 3 months.

Modification

If experiencing diarrhea, omit the onion and use 1 tablespoon onion powder. The nutrition information doesn't change.

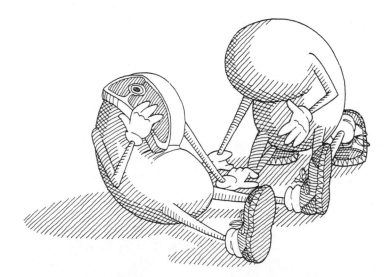

Chicken Soup

Yield: 4 servings
Preparation time: 50 minutes

2 cups chicken stock (see page 155)

1 cup canned or leftover cooked chicken, shredded

2 small, well-washed potatoes, peeled and diced

1 large, well-washed carrot, peeled and sliced

¾ cup well-washed sliced mushrooms

¼ teaspoon salt

¼ teaspoon black pepper

This traditional comfort food is a tasty way to use leftover chicken.

1. Place the stock in a large saucepan over high heat, and bring to a boil.

2. Add the chicken, vegetables, and spices, and return to a boil. Cover, reduce the heat to medium, and simmer for 25 minutes. Serve hot.

NUTRITION INFORMATION (PER SERVING):

Calories: 200   Fat: 4 g   Carbohydrate: 29 g   Protein: 13 g

Good for diarrhea, dry mouth, loss of appetite, mouth and throat sores, and nausea and vomiting.

Modification

If experiencing chewing and swallowing difficulties, pour the soup into a blender, and blend until smooth. The nutrition information doesn't change.

Easy Tomato and Rice Soup

Yield: 2 servings
Preparation time: 25 minutes

1 can (10 ½-ounces) tomato soup

½ cup low-fat milk

½ cup stock (see page 155)

⅓ cup cooked brown rice

1 tablespoon minced onion

⅛ teaspoon salt

⅛ teaspoon black pepper

This is a good use for leftover rice. If you're cooking the rice from scratch, see page 213 for instructions.

1. Place all the ingredients in a large saucepan over medium heat, and heat through. Take care that the soup doesn't boil. Serve hot.

NUTRITION INFORMATION (PER SERVING):

Calories: 235   Fat: 5 g   Carbohydrate: 40 g   Protein: 7 g

Good for alterations in taste, dry mouth, fatigue, loss of appetite, and nausea and vomiting.

Modification

If experiencing chewing and swallowing difficulties, pour the soup into a blender, and blend until smooth. The nutrition information doesn't change.

Hearty Barley Soup

Yield: 4 servings
Preparation time: 1 ½ hours

4 cups stock (see page 155)

¾ cup raw pearled barley

2 well-washed carrots, peeled
  and sliced

2 cups well-washed sliced
  mushrooms

1 well-washed tomato, chopped

1 tablespoon tomato paste

1 teaspoon salt

1 teaspoon black pepper

1 teaspoon ground paprika

1 teaspoon dried thyme

1 teaspoon dried marjoram

¼ cup vinegar

2 tablespoons chopped
  well-washed parsley

This is a thick, hearty soup with the consistency of rice pudding. On a cold fall or winter day, it is satisfying to a hungry stomach. The vinegar adds a special zing. For more information on barley, see page 168.

1. Place all the ingredients except the vinegar and parsley in a large saucepan over medium-high heat, and bring to a gentle boil. Then cover, lower the heat to medium, and simmer about 1 hour, or until the vegetables are soft and the barley is cooked.

2. Garnish each bowl with 1 tablespoon of vinegar and ½ tablespoon of parsley, and serve.

NUTRITION INFORMATION (PER SERVING):
Calories: 210   Fat: 2 g   Carbohydrate: 40 g   Protein: 10 g

Good for alterations in taste, chewing and swallowing difficulties, constipation, diarrhea, dry mouth, fatigue, loss of appetite, and nausea and vomiting.

Instant Mashed Potato Soup

Yield: 1 serving
Preparation time: 15 minutes

1 cup low-fat milk

½ cup dry instant mashed
  potatoes

¼ cup grated cheddar cheese

2 tablespoons plain low-fat
  yogurt

⅛ teaspoon salt

⅛ teaspoon black pepper

Add a slice or two of whole grain bread, and this fast-and-easy soup becomes a complete meal for one.

1. Place all the ingredients in a small saucepan over medium heat, and heat until thoroughly hot. Stir often to avoid scorching the milk. Serve immediately.

NUTRITION INFORMATION (PER SERVING):
Calories: 340   Fat: 15 g   Carbohydrate: 34 g   Protein: 19 g

Good for chewing and swallowing difficulties, dry mouth, fatigue, mouth and throat sores, and weight gain.

Lentil Soup

Yield: 4 servings
Preparation time: 2 hours

1 cup dried lentils

2 cups water

1 teaspoon canola oil

1 small onion, chopped

1 well-washed celery stalk, diced

1 well-washed carrot, sliced

1 small, well-washed potato, diced

¼ cup tomato sauce

2 cups stock (see page 155)

½ teaspoon salt

½ teaspoon black pepper

1 teaspoon garlic powder

This is a good, hearty soup that freezes well.

1. Wash the lentils, discarding any foreign material, and drain well.

2. Place the water in a large saucepan over high heat, and bring to a boil. Add the lentils, and stir once or twice. Turn off the heat, cover, and let sit for 30 minutes.

3. Place the oil in a large pot over medium heat. Add the onion and celery, and sauté until softened, about 3 minutes.

4. Add the lentils and water, and then add the remaining ingredients. Cover, and simmer about 1 hour. Serve hot.

NUTRITION INFORMATION (PER SERVING):

Calories: 140   Fat: 2 g   Carbohydrate: 25 g   Protein: 6 g

Good for alterations in taste, chewing and swallowing difficulties, constipation, dry mouth, loss of appetite, and nausea and vomiting. If fatigued, make a double batch when feeling well and freeze for up to 3 months.

Modification

If experiencing diarrhea, omit the onion and use 1 tablespoon onion powder. The nutrition information doesn't change.

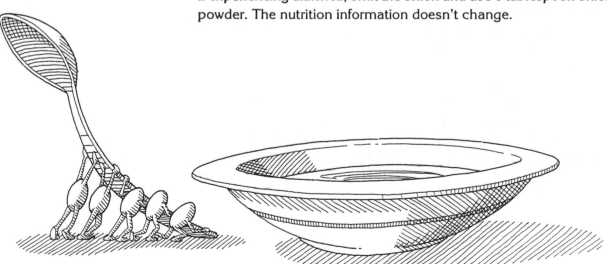

McMillan's Minestrone

Yield: 8 servings
Preparation time: 1 1/2 hours

1 cup dry couscous*

2 cups water

2 tablespoons olive oil

1 medium-sized onion, chopped

1 clove garlic, minced

1/4 cup chopped well-washed
   parsley

1/2 head well-washed cabbage,
   shredded

3 well-washed celery stalks,
   chopped

2 cups well-washed, peeled,
   and chopped turnip, zucchini,
   or potato

3 cans (14 1/2 ounces each)
   tomatoes stewed with basil
   and oregano, or plain stewed
   tomatoes to which 1
   tablespoon dried basil and 1
   tablespoon dried oregano
   have been added

2 cups garbanzo beans, cooked
   fresh or canned, rinsed and
   drained

1 cup corn kernels, thawed
   frozen or canned, drained

1 cup peas, thawed frozen or
   canned, drained

2 cups stock (see page 155)

*Couscous is a form of pasta from
the Middle East that looks like large
grains of sand.

This is a hearty soup with a mild taste. The seasonings from the canned tomato provide enough flavor, but it can't hurt to add some of your favorite herbs. Serve with Herb Bread (see page 96).

1. Place the couscous and water in a small saucepan over high heat, stir, and bring to a boil. Then cover, turn off the heat, and let sit for 5 minutes.

2. Place the oil in a large pot over medium heat. Add the onion, garlic, and parsley, and sauté for 1 minute.

3. Add the cabbage, celery, and turnip, zucchini, or potato. Stir until the vegetables are somewhat coated with the oil. Add the tomatoes, cover, and simmer until the vegetables are soft, about 15 minutes. The pot will seem very full, but it will cook down.

4. Add the garbanzo beans, corn, peas, stock, and couscous. Bring to a gentle simmer, and cook until heated thoroughly. Add stock as needed to reach the desired consistency. Serve hot, and season to taste with salt, pepper, oregano, or basil.

NUTRITION INFORMATION (PER SERVING):
Calories: 220   Fat: 6 g   Carbohydrate: 32 g   Protein: 12 g

---

Good for alterations in taste, constipation,
dry mouth, fatigue, and loss of appetite.

Potato-Zucchini Soup

Yield: 4 servings
Preparation time: 1 hour 10 minutes

2 teaspoons olive oil

2 cups chopped onion

1 clove garlic, minced

2 pounds well-washed zucchini, sliced

2 medium-sized, well-washed potatoes, sliced

2 cups stock (see page 155)

1 ½ tablespoons white or rice vinegar

4 teaspoons dried basil

½ teaspoon salt

½ teaspoon black pepper

1 cup plain low-fat yogurt

Warm or cold, this is a very comforting soup—it soothes the stomach while it sticks to the ribs. It is very soothing when served chilled and topped with yogurt if you are experiencing mouth and throat sores. Adjust the spices to your taste and tolerance.

1. Place the oil in a large pot over medium heat. Add the onion and garlic, and sauté until soft, about 3 minutes.

2. Add the zucchini, potatoes, stock, vinegar, basil, salt, and pepper. Bring the mixture to a boil over high heat, then reduce the heat to medium, cover, and simmer for 30 minutes, or until vegetables are soft. Cool the soup by placing it in the refrigerator for about 30 minutes, or until it's just warm.

3. Pour the soup into a blender in batches, and purée until smooth. If serving cold, chill in the refrigerator for 10 minutes. Garnish each bowl with ¼ cup of yogurt, and serve.

NUTRITION INFORMATION (PER SERVING):
Calories: 315   Fat: 6 g   Carbohydrate: 58 g   Protein: 12 g

---

Good for alterations in taste, chewing and swallowing difficulties, dry mouth, fatigue, mouth and throat sores, nausea and vomiting, and weight gain.

Sweet Potato Soup

Yield: 2 servings
Preparation time: 1 hour

3 large sweet potatoes, cooked,
   peeled, and coarsely chopped

2 ¾ cups stock (see page 155)

⅓ cup plain low-fat yogurt

½ cup grated Parmesan cheese

½ teaspoon black pepper

1 tablespoon soy sauce

1 teaspoon dried dill

The sweet potato is one of the most nutritious of vegetables—it's a great source of beta-carotene. If you're not sure how to cook sweet potatoes, see page 178. Or, bake them at 350°F for 1 hour.

1. Place the sweet potatoes in a blender or food processor with the stock and yogurt, and purée until smooth.

2. Place the purée in large saucepan over medium-high heat. Add the cheese, pepper, soy sauce, and dill.

3. Bring the soup to a boil, stirring often. Then reduce the heat to medium, and continue cooking until the soup thickens, about 10 to 15 minutes. Serve hot.

NUTRITION INFORMATION (PER SERVING):

Calories: 370   Fat: 10 g   Carbohydrate: 47 g   Protein: 22 g

---

Good for alterations in taste, chewing and swallowing difficulties, dry mouth, nausea and vomiting, and weight gain.

Modification

If experiencing diarrhea, omit the yogurt and cheese. Use ¾ cup light tofu and about 2 tablespoons water.

MODIFIED NUTRITION INFORMATION:

Calories: 325   Fat: 5 g   Carbohydrate: 47 g   Protein: 24 g

---

Black Bean Chili

*Yield: 6 servings
Preparation time: 3 to 3 ½
hours (after soaking beans
overnight)*

2 ½ cups dried black beans
(about 1 pound)

1 gallon water, divided

1 tablespoon olive oil

½ cup chopped onion

2 cloves garlic, minced

1 pound firm tofu, drained and
crumbled

¼ teaspoon hot sauce

2 cans (16 ounces) stewed
tomatoes, chopped

1 can (8 ounces) tomato sauce

1 can (6 ounces) tomato paste

2 tablespoons chili powder

1 teaspoon dried oregano

1 teaspoon ground cumin

1 teaspoon cayenne pepper

1 teaspoon black pepper

*This is a very tasty chili that freezes well. Serve it with rice, corn bread, or
tortillas.*

1. Rinse the beans well, then place in a large pot and cover with 8 cups
(½ gallon) of the water. Soak overnight.

2. Drain the beans, return to the pot, and cover with the remaining 8
cups of water. Cover the pot, and place over high heat. Bring to a boil,
and then reduce the heat to medium and simmer until the beans are soft,
about 1 ½ to 2 hours.

3. When the beans are soft, place the oil in an 8-inch frying pan over
medium heat. Add the onion and garlic, and sauté until soft, about 3
minutes. Add to the beans.

4. Mix the tofu, hot sauce, tomato products, and spices into the chili.
Cook for 1 hour, or until the mixture is thickened. Add additional spices
to taste just before serving.

NUTRITION INFORMATION (PER SERVING):

Calories: 450   Fat: 9 g   Carbohydrate: 70 g   Protein: 31 g

---

Good for alterations in taste, constipation, dry mouth,
loss of appetite, and weight gain. If fatigued,
make a double batch when feeling well
and freeze for up to 3 months.

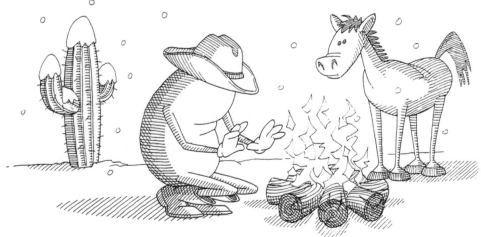

Turkey Chili

Yield: 4 servings
Preparation time: 2 hours

1 pound ground turkey

4 cloves garlic, minced

1 large onion, chopped

1 large, well-washed green bell
  pepper, seeded and chopped

1 can (15 ounces) tomato sauce

1 can (28 ounces) stewed
  tomatoes, chopped

2 cups kidney beans, cooked
  fresh or canned, rinsed and
  drained

1 tablespoon onion powder

1 tablespoon garlic powder

1 tablespoon chili powder

2 teaspoons dried oregano

1 teaspoon black pepper

1 teaspoon ground cumin

2 tablespoons soy sauce

2 teaspoons chopped
  well-washed cilantro, divided
  (optional)

The longer this chili cooks, the better. Cooking allows the flavors to blend and the chili to thicken. If you're cooking the kidney beans from scratch, see page 212.

1. Place the turkey in nonstick frying pan over medium-high heat, and cook until no longer pink. Drain off any fat.

2. Add the onion, garlic, and bell pepper. Reduce the heat to medium, and cook, covered, until the vegetables are soft, about 10 minutes.

3. Transfer the mixture to a large pot, and add the tomato sauce, tomatoes, beans, and seasonings. Simmer slowly until the seasonings blend and the chili thickens, about 45 to 60 minutes. Garnish each bowl with a ½ teaspoon of cilantro, if desired, and serve.

NUTRITION INFORMATION (PER SERVING):

Calories: 400   Fat: 10 g   Carbohydrate: 53 g   Protein: 28 g

---

Good for alterations in taste, constipation, dry mouth,
fatigue, loss of appetite, and weight gain.

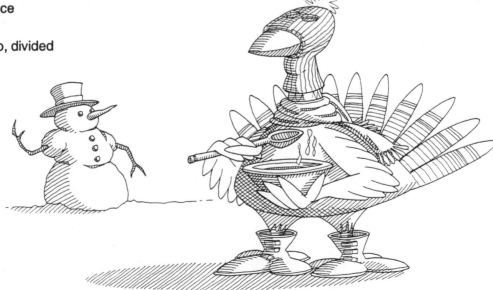

Savory Side Dishes

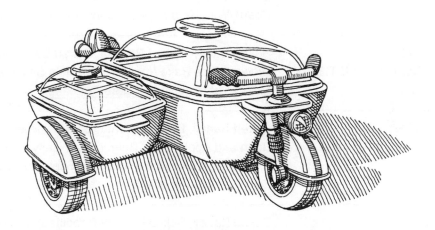

Mix and match the side dishes in this section with the entrées in the next section to create nutritionally balanced meals. You will find recipes using grains, legumes, and vegetables—all important ingredients in a healthy diet. You should also feel free to have these dishes as between-meal snacks.

Grains, such as barley, millet, and rice, are easy to store and relatively inexpensive. Once you try them, we are sure you will use them over and over again in your side dishes, soups, and entrées. They are high in complex carbohydrates and protein, and rich in both insoluble and soluble fiber. They are also a good source of B vitamins. See page 168 for directions on how to cook some of the more unusual grains, and page 213 for directions on how to cook rice.

Legumes, such as peas and dried beans, are also excellent sources of protein and fiber. We've included some tasty and easy-to-prepare legume recipes in this section. See page 212 for directions on how to cook dry legumes.

Vegetables are a must in your meal plan. They are an excellent source of vitamins and minerals. See page 178 for information on how to cook vegetables.

Recipe-by-Symptoms Chart

Different recipes in this section are designed to address different symptoms that commonly occur in people with HIV disease. This chart can help you find recipes to ease your symptoms. You'll note that some recipes address multiple symptoms.

ALTERATIONS IN TASTE

Baked Sweet Potatoes and Apples, Bean and Apple Stew, Green Beans With Herb Sauce, Spanish Rice, Zucchini Mozzarella Bake

CHEWING AND SWALLOWING DIFFICULTIES

Baked Barley, Baked Polenta, Baked Sweet Potatoes and Apples, Broccoli Rice Bake (modified), Dede's Smashed Sweet Potatoes, Millet Pilaf (modified), Potato Pancakes

CONSTIPATION

Baked Barley, Baked Polenta, Baked Sweet Potatoes and Apples, Bean and Apple Stew, Bulgur Pilaf, Easy Bean Casserole, Millet Pilaf, Rice With Spice (modified), Scalloped Corn and Tomatoes, Spanish Rice (modified)

DIARRHEA

Baked Barley, Baked Polenta (modified), Baked Sweet Potatoes and Apples, Dede's Smashed Sweet Potatoes (modified), Green Beans With Herb Sauce (modified), Potato Pancakes, Rice With Spice (modified), Scalloped Potatoes

DRY MOUTH

Baked Sweet Potatoes and Apples, Bean and Apple Stew, Broccoli Rice Bake, Dede's Smashed Sweet Potatoes, Easy Bean Casserole, Green Beans With Herb Sauce, Scalloped Corn and Tomatoes, Zucchini Mozzarella Bake

FATIGUE

Baked Barley, Baked Sweet Potatoes and Apples, Bean and Apple Stew, Broccoli Rice Bake, Dede's Smashed Sweet Potatoes, Easy Bean Casserole, Potato Pancakes, Rice With Spice, Scalloped Corn and Tomatoes, Spanish Rice, Zucchini Mozzarella Bake

LOSS OF APPETITE

Baked Barley, Baked Polenta, Baked Sweet Potatoes and Apples, Bean and Apple Stew, Bulgur Pilaf, Dede's Smashed Sweet Potatoes, Potato Pancakes, Rice With Spice, Spanish Rice

MOUTH AND THROAT SORES	Baked Barley, Baked Sweet Potatoes and Apples, Broccoli Rice Bake, Dede's Smashed Sweet Potatoes, Potato Pancakes, Rice With Spice
NAUSEA AND VOMITING	Baked Barley, Baked Polenta, Baked Sweet Potatoes and Apples, Bulgur Pilaf, Dede's Smashed Sweet Potatoes, Green Beans With Herb Sauce, Millet Pilaf, Potato Pancakes, Rice With Spice, Scalloped Potatoes
WEIGHT GAIN	Baked Sweet Potatoes and Apples, Bean and Apple Stew, Broccoli Rice Bake, Bulgur Pilaf, Dede's Smashed Sweet Potatoes, Easy Bean Casserole, Millet Pilaf, Rice With Spice, Scalloped Corn and Tomatoes, Spanish Rice, Zucchini Mozzarella Bake

Cooking Unusual Grains

Everyone is familiar with such grains as wheat, corn, and rice. But throughout history, humans have used many other grains in cooking, grains that have played—and continue to play—an important role in various cuisines around the world. We encourage you to explore cooking with these grains. Some can be found in supermarkets, while others are stocked in health food stores and gourmet shops.

Barley

Barley, one of the oldest cultivated grains, is high in soluble fiber. It has a thick outer hull than must be removed before it can be cooked. Barley can be bought either hulled, in which only the outermost layers are removed, or pearled, in which most of the outer coating is removed. Quick barley is pearled barley that has been flaked for quick cooking. Eat barley as a hot cereal, or add it to soups and casseroles. Various types of barley require various amounts of liquid and cooking times:

Per ½ cup uncooked	Liquid	Cooking Time	Serving
Hulled	2 cups	1 hour, 40 minutes	1 ¼ cup
Pearled	1 ½ cups	55 minutes	2 cups
Quick	1 cup	10 to 12 minutes	1 ½ cups

To cook barley, place the barley and the liquid in a medium-sized pot over high heat, and bring to a boil. Then reduce the heat to medium, cover, and simmer for the time shown on the chart.

Bulgur

Bulgur is wheat that has been lightly cooked, dried, and cracked. This quick-cooking and delicious grain is a staple in the Middle East and in southeastern Europe.

Bulgur can be substituted for rice in any recipe. It can be either simmered or steeped:

Simmering: Place 1 cup liquid and ½ cup bulgur in a 2-quart saucepan. Cover with a tight-fitting lid, and bring to a boil. Then reduce the heat, and simmer for 15 minutes. This makes 1 ½ cups.

Steeping: Place ½ cup bulgur in a shallow dish, and pour enough boiling liquid over it to cover by ½ inch—about 1 cup liquid. Cover the dish, and let it stand for at least 30 minutes, or until the bulgur has absorbed the liquid and softened. This makes 1 ½ cups.

Millet

Millet is a little round grain, usually ivory or yellow in color. It is an excellent source of calcium, iron, protein, and B vitamins.

Millet makes both a wonderful breakfast food and a base for many meatless dishes because it makes a good substitute for rice. To cook millet, place 1 ½ cups liquid and ½ cup of millet in a 2-quart saucepan. Cover with a tight-fitting lid, and bring to a boil. Then reduce the heat, and simmer for 25 minutes. This makes 2 ½ cups.

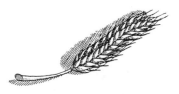

Barley

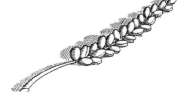

Bulgur

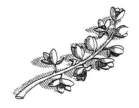

Millet

Baked Polenta

Yield: 6 servings
Preparation time: 10 minutes
to assemble; 35 to 40 minutes
to bake

13 ounces chicken stock (see
 page 155)

1 ½ cups low-fat milk

1 cup cornmeal

1 teaspoon salt

½ teaspoon white pepper

This dish is one of our tasters' favorites. Try this high-fiber Italian side dish with Black Bean Chili (page 163) or Sweet and Spicy Pork Chops (page 205).

1. Preheat the oven to 375°F.

2. Place all the ingredients in a medium-sized bowl, and mix thoroughly.

3. Coat an 8-inch square baking dish with nonstick cooking spray. Place the mixture in the dish, and bake for 35 to 40 minutes. The mixture will be very liquid to start, but will become firm as it bakes. Serve immediately.

NUTRITION INFORMATION (PER SERVING):
Calories: 110   Fat: 2 g   Carbohydrate: 19 g   Protein: 5 g

Good for chewing and swallowing difficulties, constipation,
loss of appetite, and nausea and vomiting.

Modification

If experiencing diarrhea, omit the low-fat milk, and use $1\frac{1}{2}$ cups light soymilk or lactose-reduced milk. The nutrition information doesn't change.

Baked Barley

Yield: 4 servings
Preparation time: 30 minutes to
assemble; 1 hour to bake

1 tablespoon canola oil

1 cup raw pearled barley

¼ cup chopped well-washed
 parsley

1 cup sliced well-washed
 mushrooms

3 cups heated vegetable stock,
 divided (see page 155)

Rice is nice, but if you want a nutrient-dense substitute, try barley. For more information on barley, see "Cooking Unusual Grains."

1. Preheat the oven to 350°F.

2. Place oil in a small frying pan over medium heat. Add barley and parsley, and sauté until the the barley grains are coated with oil, about 1 minute.

3. Coat an 8-inch square baking dish with nonstick cooking spray. Place the barley and parsley in the dish.

4. Sauté the mushrooms in the same frying pan until soft, about 3 minutes. Then put the mushrooms on top of the barley in the baking dish.

5. Add 2 ½ cups of stock to the baking dish, and bake, covered, at 350°F for 1 hour. Add remaining ½ cup stock during baking if necessary. Serve immediately.

NUTRITION INFORMATION (PER SERVING):

Calories: 240   Fat: 5 g   Carbohydrate: 41 g   Protein: 9 g

Good for chewing and swallowing difficulties, constipation, diarrhea, fatigue, loss of appetite, mouth and throat sores, and nausea and vomiting.

Bulgur Pilaf

Yield: 5 servings
Preparation time: 25 minutes

2 tablespoons pine nuts

1 teaspoon canola oil

1 cup chopped onion

1 cup grated well-washed carrot

1 ½ cups uncooked bulgur

½ cup currants*

1 teaspoon salt

2 cups water

*Currants are raisins made from the black corinth grape. They are seedless and very dark in color.

Bulgur gives you the flavor and nutritional value of whole wheat in a quick-cooking form. It also provides plenty of fiber. For more information on bulgur, see page 168.

1. Toast the pine nuts by placing them in a small, nonstick frying pan over medium heat, stirring constantly, until lightly brown. Set aside.

2. Place the oil in a medium-sized saucepan over medium heat. Add the onion and carrot, and sauté until tender, about 5 minutes. Add the bulgur, currants, and salt, and mix thoroughly.

3. Add the water, turn the heat to high, and bring to a boil. Then cover, reduce the heat to medium, and simmer for 10 minutes, or until the bulgur is tender and the liquid is absorbed.

4. Garnish each bowl with some pine nuts, and serve.

NUTRITION INFORMATION (PER SERVING):

Calories: 215   Fat: 3 g   Carbohydrate: 42 g   Protein: 7 g

Good for constipation, loss of appetite, nausea and vomiting, and weight gain.

Millet Pilaf

Yield: 6 servings
Preparation time: 10 minutes to assemble; 1 ½ hours to bake

1 cup whole hulled millet

2 tablespoons canola oil

2 medium-sized onions, chopped

1 well-washed carrot, sliced

1 cup sliced well-washed mushrooms

1 teaspoon salt

1 teaspoon black pepper

4 cups vegetable stock (see page 155)

1 cup plain low-fat yogurt

Millet is a better source of various B vitamins, copper, and iron than either whole wheat or brown rice. Millet's delicate and relatively bland flavor may require a little extra spice. For more information about millet, see page 168.

1. Preheat the oven to 350°F.

2. Place the millet in a large frying pan over low heat, and brown slowly, taking care to not scorch the grain. This should take about 3 minutes.

3. Add the oil and onions, and sauté until the onions are lightly browned, about 5 minutes.

4. Add the carrot, mushrooms, salt, and pepper, and cook until the carrot is tender, about 5 to 10 minutes.

5. Coat a 9-x-13-inch baking dish with nonstick cooking spray. Transfer the millet mixture to the dish.

6. Pour in the stock, and bake, tightly covered, for 1 ½ hours, or until millet is tender. You may need to add more stock during baking.

7. Garnish each serving with yogurt, and serve immediately.

NUTRITION INFORMATION (PER SERVING):
Calories: 245   Fat: 8 g   Carbohydrate: 34 g   Protein: 10 g

---

Good for constipation, nausea and vomiting, and weight gain.

Modification

If experiencing chewing and swallowing difficulties, omit the onion, and use 1 tablespoon onion powder. The nutrition information doesn't change.

Spanish Rice

Yield: 3 servings
Preparation time: 25 minutes

2 teaspoons canola oil

1 medium-sized onion, finely chopped

1 well-washed green bell pepper, seeded and finely chopped

1 ½ cups cooked white rice

1 can (6 ounces) tomato sauce

3 medium-sized, well-washed tomatoes, cubed

1 teaspoon black pepper

1 teaspoon ground cumin

1 teaspoon chili powder

This is our low-fat version of a popular side dish. See page 213 for instructions on how to cook rice.

1. Place the oil in a large frying pan over medium heat. Add the onion and green pepper, and sauté until tender, about 5 minutes.

2. Add the remaining ingredients, and cook 10 more minutes, or until the vegetables are tender-crisp. Serve immediately.

NUTRITION INFORMATION (PER SERVING):

Calories: 220   Fat: 4 g   Carbohydrate: 44 g   Protein: 5 g

Good for alterations in taste, fatigue,
loss of appetite, and weight gain.

Modification

If experiencing constipation, omit the white rice, and use brown rice.

MODIFIED NUTRITION INFORMATION:

Calories: 206   Fat: 5 g   Carbohydrate: 39 g   Protein: 5 g

Rice With Spice

Yield: 4 servings
Preparation time: 25 to 30 minutes

1 cup uncooked white rice

2 cups water

½ cup raisins

2 teaspoons ground cinnamon

1 teaspoon salt

For a change of pace, try this dish cold with a spoonful of low-fat plain yogurt on top.

1. Place all the ingredients in a large saucepan, and place over high heat. Bring to a boil, then cover and cook over medium-low heat for 20 to 25 minutes, or until the rice is done. Serve immediately, or place in an airtight container and store for up to 3 days in the refrigerator.

NUTRITION INFORMATION (PER SERVING):

Calories: 230   Fat: 1 g   Carbohydrate: 54 g   Protein: 4 g

Good for fatigue, loss of appetite, mouth and throat sores,
nausea and vomiting, and weight gain.

Modifications

If experiencing diarrhea, omit the raisins, and mix $\frac{1}{2}$ cup canned fruit with the cooked rice.

MODIFIED NUTRITION INFORMATION:

Calories: 195   Fat: 1 g   Carbohydrate: 44 g   Protein: 3 g

If experiencing constipation, omit the white rice and water, and use brown rice and 2 $\frac{1}{2}$ cups of water. Cook for 45 to 50 minutes.

MODIFIED NUTRITION INFORMATION:

Calories: 200   Fat: 1 g   Carbohydrates: 45 g   Protein: 3 g

---

Potato Pancakes

Yield: 12 pancakes
Preparation time: 30 minutes

4 egg whites

1 tablespoon white flour

$\frac{1}{2}$ teaspoon salt

$\frac{1}{4}$ tablespoon ground nutmeg

2 cups peeled and grated well-washed potato (2 large potatoes)

Potato pancakes are a high-energy food. Our resident expert advises that you serve them with a cup of English Breakfast tea and The New York Times.

1. Coat a griddle with nonstick cooking spray, and preheat over medium heat.

2. Place all the ingredients in a large bowl, and mix thoroughly.

3. Spoon $\frac{1}{4}$ cup batter per pancake onto the griddle, flatten with a fork, and cook on both sides until lightly browned—about 3 minutes a side. Serve with warmed applesauce, plain low-fat yogurt, or your favorite fruit.

NUTRITION INFORMATION (PER 3-PANCAKE SERVING):

Calories: 150   Fat: less than 1 g   Carbohydrate: 32 g   Protein: 6 g

---

Good for chewing and swallowing difficulties, diarrhea,
fatigue, loss of appetite, mouth and throat sores,
and nausea and vomiting.

Dede's Smashed Sweet Potatoes

Yield: 4 servings
Preparation time: 40 minutes

2 medium-sized, well-washed
   sweet potatoes, cut into
   pieces

2 medium-sized, well-washed
   white potatoes, cut into
   pieces

½ cup low-fat cottage cheese

½ cup evaporated skim milk

¼ cup nonfat dry milk powder

½ teaspoon salt

1 teaspoon black pepper

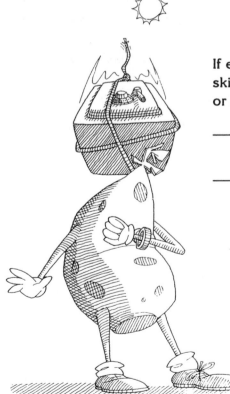

This recipe adds a flavor twist to a favorite comfort food.

1. Place the potatoes in a large saucepan over high heat, and cover with water. Boil for 15 minutes, or until tender. Drain.

2. Place the potatoes and the remaining ingredients in a large bowl, and beat with an electric mixer until smooth. You can also mash the potatoes by hand, using either a potato masher or a large spoon. Serve immediately.

NUTRITION INFORMATION (PER SERVING):

Calories: 180   Fat: 1 g   Carbohydrate: 34 g   Protein: 10 g

---

Good for chewing and swallowing difficulties, dry mouth,
fatigue, loss of appetite, mouth and throat sores,
nausea and vomiting, and weight gain.

Modification

If experiencing diarrhea, omit the cottage cheese and evaporated skim milk, and use 1 cup light, drained tofu and ½ cup light soymilk or lactose-reduced milk. Remove the potato skins.

MODIFIED NUTRITION INFORMATION:

Calories: 265   Fat: 3 g   Carbohydrate: 45 g   Protein: 17 g

---

Baked Sweet Potatoes and Apples

Yield: 4 servings
Preparation time: 5 minutes to assemble; 45 minutes to bake

2 cooked sweet potatoes, peeled and cubed, or 1 can (16 ounces) of sweet potatoes

½ cup light soymilk

1 jar (16 ounces) applesauce

2 tablespoons brown sugar

1 tablespoon ground cinnamon

1 teaspoon ground nutmeg

Sweet potatoes aren't just for holidays! Try this comforting recipe all year round. You can steam or microwave the sweet potatoes (see page 178). Or bake them at 350°F for 1 hour.

1. Preheat the oven to 375°F.

2. Coat an 8-inch square baking dish with nonstick cooking spray. Place all the ingredients in the dish, and mix thoroughly. Cover, and bake for 45 minutes, or until heated through. Serve immediately.

NUTRITION INFORMATION (PER SERVING):
Calories: 335   Fat: 1 g   Carbohydrate: 82 g   Protein: 5 g

Good for all symptoms.

Bean and Apple Stew

Yield: 2 servings
Preparation time: 10 minutes to assemble; 15 minutes to cook

1 can (16 ounces) baked beans

1 tablespoon molasses

1 tablespoon vinegar

1 tablespoon prepared mustard

1 large, well-washed apple, cored and chopped

Take that can of baked beans and spice it up!

1. Place all the ingredients in a medium-sized saucepan over medium heat, and mix thoroughly. Cover, and simmer for at least 15 minutes, or until heated through. Serve immediately.

NUTRITION INFORMATION (PER SERVING):
Calories: 280   Fat: 1 g   Carbohydrate: 63 g   Protein: 12 g

Good for alterations in taste, constipation, dry mouth, fatigue, loss of appetite, and weight gain.

Scalloped Potatoes

Yield: 6 servings
Preparation time: 10 minutes to assemble; 1 hour to bake

2 tablespoons white flour

1 teaspoon salt

1 teaspoon black pepper

3 well-washed potatoes, peeled and sliced

1 tablespoon margarine

1 ½ cups light soymilk

1 cup bread crumbs

1 teaspoon ground paprika

Often, scalloped potatoes are loaded with fat. We designed this recipe to be low-fat—and still taste great!

1. Preheat the oven to 400°F.

2. Place the flour, salt, and pepper in a small bowl, and mix thoroughly.

3. Coat a 9-x-13-inch baking dish with nonstick cooking spray. Arrange a third of the potatoes on the bottom of the dish. Sprinkle a third of the flour mixture over the potatoes, and dot with a third of the margarine. Add two more layers, for a total of three layers.

4. Pour the soymilk over the potatoes, and top with the bread crumbs and paprika. Bake for 1 hour, or until the potatoes are soft when pierced with a fork. Serve immediately.

NUTRITION INFORMATION (PER SERVING):
Calories: 200   Fat: 2 g   Carbohydrate: 40 g   Protein: 5 g

Good for diarrhea, and nausea and vomiting.

Scalloped Corn and Tomatoes

Yield: 6 servings
Preparation time: 10 minutes to assemble; 20 minutes to bake

2 tablespoons canola oil

4 well-washed tomatoes, sliced thickly

1 can (15 ounces) corn kernels, drained

1 cup bread crumbs

¼ cup butter

Serve this dish with your favorite chicken recipe.

1. Preheat the oven to 350°F.

2. Coat a 9-x-13-inch baking dish with nonstick cooking spray. Spread the tomatoes on the bottom of the dish. Pour the corn over the tomatoes.

3. Top the corn with the bread crumbs, and dot with the butter. Bake for about 20 minutes, or until the crumbs are toasted. Serve immediately.

NUTRITION INFORMATION (PER SERVING):
Calories: 185   Fat: 12 g   Carbohydrate: 18 g   Protein: 3 g

---

Good for constipation, dry mouth, fatigue, and weight gain.

Broccoli Rice Bake

Yield: 4 servings
Preparation time: 15 minutes to assemble; 30 minutes to bake

1 package (10 ounces) frozen chopped broccoli, thawed and drained

¼ cup chopped onion

1 ½ cups cooked brown rice

¾ cup shredded cheddar cheese

3 eggs

½ teaspoon salt

¼ cup low-fat milk

1 teaspoon black pepper

Broccoli is a good source of beta-carotene and vitamin C. If you are cooking the rice from scratch, see page 213 for directions.

1. Preheat the oven to 350°F.

2. Place all the ingredients in a large bowl, and mix thoroughly.

3. Coat a 9-inch square baking dish with nonstick cooking spray. Pour the mixture into the dish, cover, and bake for 30 minutes, or until heated through. Serve immediately.

NUTRITION INFORMATION (PER SERVING):

Calories: 240   Fat: 12 g   Carbohydrate: 21 g   Protein: 13 g

---

Good for dry mouth, fatigue, mouth and throat sores, and weight gain.

Modification

If experiencing chewing and swallowing difficulties, omit the onion. The nutrition information doesn't change.

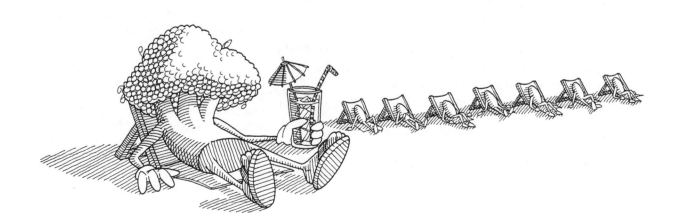

Easy Bean Casserole

Yield: 4 servings
Preparation time: 10 minutes to assemble; 20 minutes to bake

1 package (10 ounces) frozen green beans, thawed and drained

1 can (15 ounces) cream of mushroom soup

2 cups commercially prepared French fried onions

This quick recipe is also quite tasty. Green beans are a good source of beta-carotene and vitamin C.

1. Preheat the oven to 325°F.

2. Place the beans and soup in a medium-sized bowl, and mix thoroughly.

3. Coat a pie pan or an 8-inch square baking dish with nonstick cooking spray. Spoon the bean mixture into the pan or dish, and top with the onions. Cover, and bake for 20 minutes, or until heated through. Serve immediately.

NUTRITION INFORMATION (PER SERVING):
Calories: 245   Fat: 14 g   Carbohydrate: 26 g   Protein: 5 g

Good for constipation, dry mouth, fatigue, and weight gain.

Cooking Vegetables

The nutritional content of vegetables is affected by the way they are stored, handled, and—especially—cooked. In general, vegetables should be cooked with a minimum of liquid, or none at all, until they are barely tender. Potatoes, of course, are the exception. It's also important to serve cooked vegetables promptly because the longer they stand, whether in the refrigerator or at room temperature, the higher their nutrient losses.

The old days of boiling vegetables until they were limp and unappetizing are gone! There are three nutritious ways to cook vegetables: steaming, stir-frying, and microwaving.

Steaming

Steamed vegetables are delicious with a little butter, some grated cheese, and seasonings such as oregano, basil, pepper, lemon pepper, or garlic powder. To steam vegetables:

1. Wash the vegetables thoroughly, and cut to the desired size.

2. Put ½ inch of water in the bottom of a saucepan. Cover with a tight-fitting lid, and bring to a boil. Add the vegetables, either in a steamer basket or as is, and cover tightly. Or use a specially designed steamer—see the housewares section of your local department store.

Zucchini Mozzarella Bake

Yield: 4 servings
Preparation time: 10 minutes
to assemble; 20 to 25 minutes
to bake

1 cup tomato sauce

½ teaspoon salt

1 teaspoon black pepper

1 teaspoon dried oregano

1 teaspoon dried basil

2 large, well-washed zucchini, sliced

1 cup shredded mozzarella cheese

This dish is a tasty alternative to traditional lasagna. Serve with Herb Bread (page 96).

1. Preheat the oven to 325°F.

2. Place the tomato sauce, salt, pepper, oregano, and basil in a small bowl, and mix thoroughly.

3. Coat an 8-inch square baking dish with nonstick cooking spray. Place alternating layers of zucchini, cheese, and tomato sauce in the dish. Bake, uncovered, for 20 to 25 minutes, or until the zucchini is soft when pierced with a fork. Serve immediately.

NUTRITION INFORMATION (PER SERVING):

Calories: 220   Fat: 15 g   Carbohydrate: 10 g   Protein: 15 g

---

Good for alterations in taste, dry mouth, fatigue, and weight gain.

---

3. Cook over medium heat until tender-crisp, usually about 5 to 10 minutes depending upon the size and thickness of the pieces. Drain.

Stir-frying

To increase the flavor, try adding ginger, garlic, soy sauce, tamari sauce, nuts, or spices to the vegetables as they cook. To stir-fry vegetables:

1. Wash the vegetables thoroughly, and cut to the desired size. Cutting the vegetables diagonally will increase their surface area, and thus allow for faster cooking times.

2. Heat a wok or frying pan over high heat. Add 1 to 3 teaspoons of oil.

3. Add the vegetables. Cook, stirring frequently, until they are tender-crisp, about 2 to 5 minutes. If you are cooking several different types of

vegetables at once, begin cooking the largest and thickest types first, and add the remaining smaller pieces after about 2 minutes. Don't overcrowd the pan.

Microwaving

Microwaving is a very good vegetable-cooking option because it is a quick, waterless method, which allows for a high retention of nutrients. To microwave vegetables:

1. Wash the vegetables thoroughly, and cut into bite-sized pieces.

2. Place the vegetable pieces on a microwave-safe plate, and cover them with microwave-safe plastic wrap.

3. Microwave until tender-crisp, about 3 to 5 minutes.

Green Beans With Herb Sauce

Yield: 6 servings
Preparation time: 20 minutes

2 packages (10 ounces each) frozen French-style green beans, cooked per package directions

1 tablespoon butter

1 small onion, minced

2 tablespoons minced well-washed parsley

1 teaspoon dried thyme, or 1 tablespoon chopped fresh

3 tablespoons lemon juice, preferably fresh-squeezed

½ teaspoon salt

1 teaspoon black pepper

1 teaspoon ground paprika

Dress up your green beans with this flavorful, easy-to-prepare sauce.

1. Place the beans in a serving dish.

2. Place the butter in a medium-sized skillet over medium heat. Add the onions, and sauté until soft, about 3 minutes. Add the remaining ingredients, and heat through.

3. Pour the mixture over the green beans. Serve immediately.

NUTRITION INFORMATION (PER SERVING):

Calories: 55   Fat: 2 g   Carbohydrate: 9 g   Protein: 2 g

Good for alterations in taste, dry mouth,
and nausea and vomiting.

Modification

If experiencing diarrhea, omit the onion, and use 2 tablespoons onion powder.

MODIFIED NUTRITION INFORMATION:

Calories: 50   Fat: 2 g   Carbohydrate: 8 g   Protein: 2 g

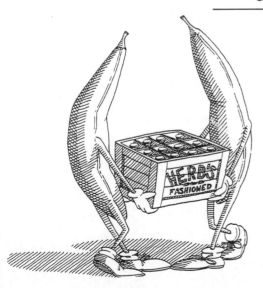

Main Fare

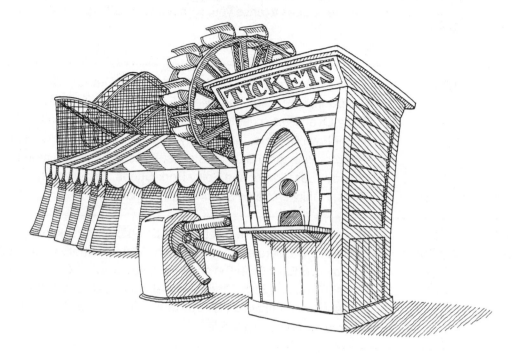

Many of the recipes in this section are comfort foods we remembered from our growing up. Comfort foods are those recipes that provide you with soothing memories and nourishing thoughts as well as healthy ingredients. These recipes— for poultry, fish, and meat—tend to be easy to prepare, and they call for ingredients found in most kitchens.

Although some of these recipes may contain canned ingredients to simplify preparation, we encourage you to use fresh ingredients whenever possible. (For information on cooking fresh vegetables, see page 178.) It's also best to use the lean meats, such as skinned chicken and turkey, to maximize protein content while limiting fat.

When planning your main meals, choose side dishes that will round out your daily requirements (see page 165). Include a protein food, a complex carbohydrate food, and a vegetable. For example, serve rice and steamed broccoli with Easy Oven Barbecue. Some recipes, such as casseroles, provide everything in one dish.

We hope you will find some of your favorite comfort foods on the following pages, or will develop a taste for some of ours.

Recipe-by-Symptoms Chart

Different recipes in this section are designed to address different symptoms that commonly occur in people with HIV disease. This chart can help you find recipes to ease your symptoms. You'll note that some recipes address multiple symptoms.

ALTERATIONS IN TASTE	Baked Parmesan Fish Fillets, Chicken à la Orange, Chicken Tandoori, Cornmeal Fish Fillets, Easy Chicken Teriyaki, Easy Oven Barbecue, Hamburger Noodle Feast, Hawaiian Chicken, Hometown Burgers, Lemon-Soy Chicken, Mediterranean Baked Shrimp, Pineapple Salmon Steaks, Poached Fish, Salmon Loaf, Sloppy Joes, Sweet and Spicy Pork Chops, Tamale Pie, Toasty Chicken Salad Sandwiches, Tuna Bake
CHEWING AND SWALLOWING DIFFICULTIES	Baked Parmesan Fish Fillets, Beef Stroganoff, Chicken and Artichoke Casserole, Cornmeal Fish Fillets, Hometown Burgers, Microwave Easy Crab Delight, Mini Meat Loaves, Oven Meatballs, Pacific Steamed Fish, Pineapple Salmon Steaks, Poached Fish, Salmon Loaf (modified), Sloppy Joes, Tuna Bake, Turkey à la King, Turkey and Rice Casserole
CONSTIPATION	Cornmeal Fish Fillets (modified), Hamburger Noodle Feast, Mexican Baked Chicken With Beans, Mini Meat Loaves, Tamale Pie, Turkey and Rice Casserole, Turkey Burger
DIARRHEA	Easy Chicken Teriyaki, Lemon-Soy Chicken, Oven Fried Scallops, Oven Meatballs, Pacific Steamed Fish (modified), Poached Fish (modified), Sloppy Joes (modified)
DRY MOUTH	Beef Stroganoff, Chicken and Artichoke Casserole, Hamburger Noodle Feast, Microwave Easy Crab Delight, Mini Meat Loaves, Oven Meatballs, Pineapple Salmon Steaks, Salmon Loaf, Sloppy Joes, Toasty Chicken Salad Sandwiches, Tuna Bake, Turkey à la King, Turkey and Rice Casserole

FATIGUE

Baked Parmesan Fish Fillets, Easy Chicken Teriyaki, Easy Oven Barbecue, Lemon-Soy Chicken, Mexican Baked Chicken With Beans, Microwave Easy Crab Delight, Mini Meat Loaves, Oven Fried Chicken, Pacific Steamed Fish, Pineapple Salmon Steaks, Pork Chop Baked With Apples and Sweet Potatoes, Sloppy Joes, Sweet and Spicy Pork Chops, Tamale Pie, Toasty Chicken Salad Sandwiches, Tuna Bake, Turkey à la King, Turkey and Rice Casserole, Turkey Burger

LOSS OF APPETITE

Chicken à la Orange, Chicken and Artichoke Casserole, Chicken Tandoori, Cornmeal Fish Fillets, Easy Chicken Teriyaki, Lemon-Soy Chicken, Mediterranean Baked Shrimp, Mini Meat Loaves, Oven Fried Chicken, Oven Fried Scallops, Oven Meatballs, Pacific Steamed Fish, Pineapple Salmon Steaks, Poached Fish, Pork Chop Baked With Apples and Sweet Potatoes, Sweet and Spicy Pork Chops

MOUTH AND THROAT SORES

Beef Stroganoff, Chicken and Artichoke Casserole, Microwave Easy Crab Delight (modified), Mini Meat Loaves, Oven Meatballs, Salmon Loaf (modified), Turkey à la King, Turkey and Rice Casserole

NAUSEA AND VOMITING

Chicken à la Orange, Easy Chicken Teriyaki, Lemon-Soy Chicken, Oven Fried Chicken, Oven Fried Scallops, Oven Meatballs, Pacific Steamed Fish, Pineapple Salmon Steaks, Poached Fish, Pork Chop Baked With Apples and Sweet Potatoes, Sloppy Joes (modified)

WEIGHT GAIN

Baked Parmesan Fish Fillets, Beef Stroganoff, Chicken and Artichoke Casserole, Chicken Tandoori, Cornmeal Fish Fillets, Hamburger Noodle Feast, Hawaiian Chicken, Hometown Burgers, Mediterranean Baked Shrimp, Mexican Baked Chicken With Beans, Microwave Easy Crab Delight, Salmon Loaf, Sloppy Joes, Tamale Pie, Toasty Chicken Salad Sandwiches, Tuna Bake, Turkey à la King, Turkey and Rice Casserole, Turkey Burger

Easy Oven Barbecue

Yield: 4 servings
Preparation time: 5 minutes to assemble; 45 to 50 minutes to bake

1 ½ pounds chicken pieces, skinned, rinsed, and dried

1 cup barbecue sauce, prepared or homemade

HOMEMADE BARBECUE SAUCE

1 tablespoon brown sugar

2 tablespoons Worcestershire sauce

1 tablespoon vinegar

¼ cup catsup

You don't need a grill and a hot summer day to enjoy barbecue!

1. Preheat the oven to 375°F.

2. Coat a 9-x-13-inch baking dish with nonstick cooking spray. Arrange the chicken pieces, meaty side up, in the dish.

3. If making the homemade sauce, place all of the ingredients in a small bowl, and mix thoroughly.

4. Brush the chicken liberally with the sauce. Bake, uncovered, for 45 to 50 minutes, or until the juices run clear when the chicken is pierced with a fork. Serve immediately.

NUTRITION INFORMATION (PER SERVING):

Calories: 135   Fat: 3 g   Carbohydrate: 5 g   Protein: 18 g

Good for alterations in taste and fatigue.

Chicken à la Orange

Yield: 4 servings
Preparation time: 15 minutes to assemble; 45 minutes to bake

1 egg, slightly beaten

¼ cup orange juice

1 cup bread crumbs

1 teaspoon ground paprika

1 teaspoon salt

1 tablespoon grated orange peel

1 ½ pounds chicken pieces, skinned, rinsed, and dried

Chicken and citrus go well together, and this dish proves it.

1. Preheat the oven to 375°F.

2. Place the egg and orange juice in a medium-sized bowl, and beat together.

3. Place the bread crumbs, paprika, salt, and orange peel in another medium-sized bowl, and mix thoroughly.

4. Dip each chicken piece in the egg mixture, and then in the bread crumb mixture.

5. Coat a 9-x-13-inch baking dish with nonstick cooking spray. Place the chicken in the dish. Bake, covered, for 30 minutes. Uncover, and bake another 15 minutes. Serve immediately.

Easy Chicken Teriyaki

*Yield: 4 servings
Preparation time: 5 minutes
to assemble; 45 to 50 minutes
to bake*

½ cup teriyaki sauce

½ cup chicken stock (see page 155)

½ cup white vinegar

½ teaspoon garlic powder

¼ teaspoon ground ginger

4 chicken breast halves, skinned, rinsed, and dried

Serve with steamed rice and cooked carrots for a complete meal.

1. Preheat the oven to 375°F.

2. Place all the ingredients except the chicken in a 9-x-13-inch baking dish, and mix thoroughly.

3. Add the chicken pieces, and turn a few times to coat with the sauce. Arrange so that the fleshy side of the chicken is on the bottom.

4. Bake, covered, for 45 to 50 minutes, or until the juices run clear when the chicken is pierced with a fork. Serve immediately.

Microwave Cooking

Place all the ingredients except the chicken in a microwave-safe baking dish, and mix thoroughly. Add the chicken pieces, turning a few times to coat with sauce, and arrange so that the meatier parts are toward the edge of the dish. Cover with wax paper, and microwave on high power for 18 to 20 minutes, rotating the dish a half turn after 9 to 10 minutes. When cooked through, keep covered and let stand 4 minutes before serving.

Hawaiian Chicken

Yield: 6 servings
Preparation time: 20 minutes
to assemble; 45 to 50 minutes
to bake

½ cup white flour

1 teaspoon ground paprika

½ teaspoon salt

¼ teaspoon black pepper

2 ½ pounds chicken pieces,
   skinned, rinsed, and dried

2 tablespoons canola oil

1 can (6 ounces) crushed
   pineapple, in water or juice

Grated rind of 1 orange

⅔ cup orange juice

In this recipe, the spices and the sweet fruit flavors work together in a delightful manner to spark your taste buds.

1. Preheat the oven to 375°F.

2. Place the flour, paprika, salt, and pepper in a large bowl, and mix thoroughly. Coat the chicken with the flour mixture.

3. Place the oil in a frying pan over medium-high heat. Add the chicken, and brown on both sides, about 2 minutes a side.

4. Place the chicken in a 9-x-13-inch baking dish, meaty side up. Add the pineapple and its juice, and the orange rind and juice. Bake, covered, for 30 to 35 minutes. Remove the lid, and bake an additional 15 minutes, or until the juices run clear when the chicken is pierced with a fork. Serve immediately.

NUTRITION INFORMATION (PER SERVING):

Calories: 330   Fat: 11 g   Carbohydrate: 20 g   Protein: 36 g

Good for alterations in taste and weight gain.

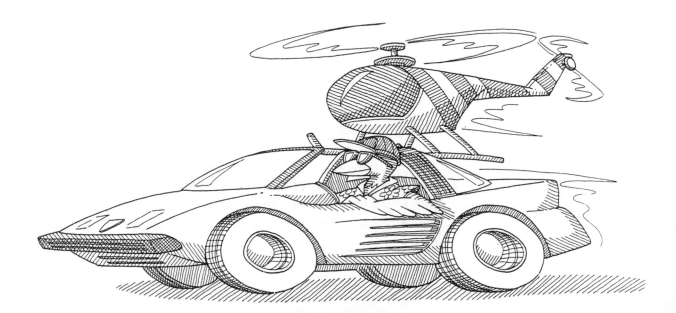

Chicken and Artichoke Casserole

Yield: 4 servings
Preparation time: 20 minutes to assemble; 40 minutes to bake

1 ½ pounds chicken pieces, skinned, rinsed, and dried

1 teaspoon salt

¼ teaspoon black pepper

½ teaspoon ground paprika

3 tablespoons butter, divided

¼ pound well-washed mushrooms, cut into large pieces

2 tablespoons white flour

⅔ cup chicken stock (see page 155)

1 can (15 ounces) artichoke hearts, drained

For a sumptuous feast, try serving this dish with Baked Sweet Potatoes and Apples (see page 175).

1. Preheat the oven to 375°F.

2. Dust the chicken pieces with the salt, pepper, and paprika.

3. Place two tablespoons of the butter in a large frying pan over medium-high heat, and brown the chicken pieces, about 2 minutes a side. Place the pieces in a 9-x-13-inch baking dish.

4. Place the other tablespoon of butter in a medium-sized frying pan over medium heat. Add the mushrooms, and sauté until they are soft, about 5 minutes. Sprinkle the flour over the mushrooms, and pour in the broth. Simmer for 5 minutes.

5. Arrange the artichoke hearts between the chicken pieces, and pour the mushroom sauce over the chicken. Cover, and bake for 40 minutes, or until the juice runs clear when the chicken is pierced with a fork. Serve immediately.

NUTRITION INFORMATION (PER SERVING):

Calories: 365   Fat: 18 g   Carbohydrate: 14 g   Protein: 38 g

---

Good for chewing and swallowing difficulties, dry mouth,
loss of appetite, mouth and throat sores, and weight gain.

Chicken Tandoori

Yield: 4 servings
Preparation time: 15 minutes to assemble; 24 hours to marinate; 40 to 50 minutes to bake

1 cup plain low-fat yogurt

3 tablespoons lime juice

1 ½ teaspoons grated fresh ginger root, or ½ teaspoon ground ginger

1 ½ teaspoons ground coriander

1 teaspoon ground cumin

½ teaspoon ground anise seeds

½ teaspoon ground cayenne pepper

1 clove garlic, finely chopped

1 ½ pounds chicken pieces, skinned, rinsed, and dried

⅓ cup butter, melted

Lime wedges

This is a great dish for when you want to impress your friends with your culinary tastes. Don't forget to marinate the chicken overnight—that allows the spices to blend.

1. Place all of the ingredients—except the chicken, butter, and lime wedges—in a medium-sized bowl, and mix thoroughly.

2. Place the chicken in a large bowl, and pour the yogurt mixture over chicken. Cover, and marinate in the refrigerator for 24 hours, turning often.

3. Preheat the oven to 375°F.

4. Place the chicken pieces in a 9-x-13-inch baking dish, and bake for 40 to 50 minutes, or until the juices run clear when the chicken is pierced with a fork. Brush with the melted butter during cooking. Serve with the lime wedges.

NUTRITION INFORMATION (PER SERVING):
Calories: 305   Fat: 18 g   Carbohydrate: 7 g   Protein: 29 g

---

Good for alterations in taste, loss of appetite, and weight gain.

Lemon-Soy Chicken

Yield: 2 servings
Preparation time: 10 minutes to assemble; 45 to 50 minutes to bake

½ cup soy sauce

½ cup lemon juice

2 chicken breasts, skinned, rinsed, and dried

This dish is so simple but so good!

1. Preheat the oven to 375°F.

2. Place the soy sauce and lemon juice in a 8-inch square baking dish, and mix thoroughly.

3. Place the chicken in the pan, meaty side up. Spoon the soy and lemon mixture on top of the chicken. Bake, covered, for 30 minutes. Remove the lid, and bake an additional 15 to 20 minutes, or until the juices run clear when the chicken is pierced with a fork.

4. Baste the chicken before placing it on the serving platter. Serve immediately.

NUTRITION INFORMATION (PER SERVING):

Calories: 195   Fat: 3 g   Carbohydrate: 10 g   Protein: 30 g

---

Good for alterations in taste, diarrhea, fatigue,
loss of appetite, and nausea and vomiting.

Mexican Baked Chicken With Beans

Yield: 4 servings
Preparation time: 5 minutes
to assemble; 45 to 50 minutes
to bake

2 cans (16 ounces each) pinto
  beans, rinsed and drained

1 ½ pounds chicken pieces,
  skinned, rinsed, and dried

1 cup prepared salsa

1 cup shredded cheddar cheese

1 avocado

Spicy salsa and mild avocado combine to give this dish a flavor all its own.

1. Preheat the oven to 375°F.

2. Place the beans in a 9-x-13-inch baking dish. Place the chicken on top of the beans, and cover with the salsa.

3. Bake, covered, for 45 to 50 minutes, or until the juices run clear when the chicken is pierced with a fork. Sprinkle the cheese on top, and allow it to melt, about 2 minutes.

4. When the chicken is almost done, peel, pit, and slice the avocado. Top the chicken with the avocado slices just before serving.

NUTRITION INFORMATION (PER SERVING):

Calories: 610   Fat: 27 g   Carbohydrate: 40 g   Protein: 54 g

---

Good for constipation, fatigue, and weight gain.

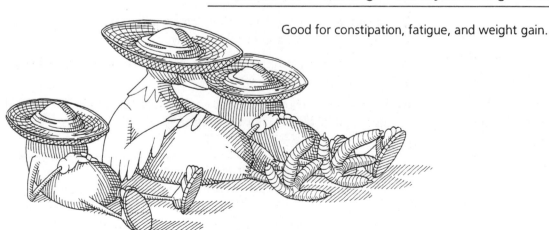

Oven Fried Chicken

Yield: 4 servings
Preparation time: 15 minutes to assemble; 45 to 50 minutes to bake

1 cup crushed corn flakes

¼ teaspoon ground paprika

¼ teaspoon onion powder

¼ teaspoon garlic powder

¼ cup low-fat milk

4 boneless chicken breast halves, skinned, rinsed, and dried

Want the flavor of fried chicken without the fat? Try this recipe.

1. Preheat the oven to 375°F.

2. Place corn flakes and spices in a medium-sized bowl, and mix thoroughly. Place the milk in another medium-sized bowl. Dip the chicken in the milk, and then in the corn flake mixture. Make sure the chicken is well coated.

3. Coat a 9-x-13-inch baking dish with nonstick cooking spray. Place the chicken in the dish, and bake, uncovered, for 45 to 50 minutes, or until the juices run clear when the chicken is pierced with a fork. Serve immediately.

NUTRITION INFORMATION (PER SERVING):
Calories: 200   Fat: 3 g   Carbohydrate: 12 g   Protein: 28 g

---

Good for fatigue, loss of appetite, and nausea and vomiting.

Toasty Chicken Salad Sandwiches

Yield: 2 servings
Preparation time: 15 minutes to assemble; 12 to 15 minutes to bake

1 cup cubed cooked chicken

½ cup diced well-washed celery

2 teaspoons minced onion

2 teaspoons lemon juice

⅓ cup plain low-fat yogurt

1 teaspoon ground paprika

2 slices bread

These open-faced sandwiches give you a tasty way to use leftover baked chicken.

1. Preheat the oven to 400°F.

2. Place the chicken, celery, onion, lemon juice, yogurt, and paprika in a medium-sized bowl, and mix thoroughly.

3. Place a scoop of chicken salad on each piece of bread, and spread the salad to form an even layer.

4. Place the bread on a nonstick cookie sheet, and bake for 12 to 15 minutes, or until bubbly. Serve immediately.

NUTRITION INFORMATION (PER SERVING):
Calories: 270   Fat: 5 g   Carbohydrate: 16 g   Protein: 38 g

---

Good for alterations in taste, dry mouth, fatigue, and weight gain.

Turkey Burger

Yield: 1 burger
Preparation time: 17 minutes

6 ounces ground turkey

1 egg

½ cup oat bran

¼ teaspoon salt

¼ teaspoon black pepper

1 whole wheat bun

This burger is very tasty all on its own, but you can build on the flavors by topping it with cranberry sauce.

1. Place all the ingredients except the bun in a small bowl, and mix thoroughly. Shape the turkey mixture into a patty.

2. Place the patty in a nonstick frying pan over medium heat, and cook until well done, about 12 minutes. Serve immediately on the bun.

NUTRITION INFORMATION (PER PATTY):

Calories: 495   Fat: 22 g   Carbohydrate: 51 g   Protein: 40 g

---

Good for constipation, fatigue, and weight gain.

Turkey à la King

Yield: 4 servings
Preparation time: 15 minutes
to assemble; 20 to 30 minutes
to cook

3 cups diced cooked turkey

1 can (3 oz.) sliced mushrooms

½ cup peas, thawed frozen or canned, drained

½ cup carrots, thawed frozen or canned, drained

¼ cup chopped pimiento

1 can (10 ¾ oz.) condensed cream of chicken soup

1 cup low-fat milk

¼ teaspoon salt

¼ teaspoon black pepper

8 slices bread

We use mushrooms, peas, and carrots in this recipe, but you can use other vegetables, such as zucchini or broccoli.

1. Place all the ingredients except the bread in a large saucepan over medium heat, and cook for 20 to 30 minutes, stirring occasionally.

2. Serve immediately over the bread (toasted or untoasted), 2 slices a serving.

NUTRITION INFORMATION (PER SERVING):

Calories: 490   Fat: 14 g   Carbohydrate: 47 g   Protein: 43 g

---

Good for chewing and swallowing difficulties (use soft bread), dry mouth, fatigue, mouth and throat sores, and weight gain.

Turkey and Rice Casserole

Yield: 4 servings
Preparation time: 15 minutes to assemble; 1 hour to bake

1 pound ground turkey

2 cups uncooked white rice

4 cups water

2 cans (10 ¾ ounces each) condensed cream of mushroom soup

1 package dry onion soup mix

Casseroles are the ultimate time savers and can be completely satisfying. Try different canned or packaged soups to alter the flavor, and add your favorite vegetables if your symptoms allow.

1. Preheat the oven to 350°F.

2. Place turkey in a nonstick frying pan over medium heat, and cook until meat is no longer pink, about 10 minutes. Drain any grease that accumulates.

3. Place turkey in a 9-x-13-inch baking dish, and sprinkle with the rice.

4. Place the water, soup, and onion mix in a medium-sized bowl, and mix thoroughly. Pour into the baking dish. Cover the dish, and bake for 1 hour, or until the rice is tender and fluid is absorbed. Serve immediately.

NUTRITION INFORMATION (PER SERVING):
Calories: 590   Fat: 12 g   Carbohydrate: 83 g   Protein: 36 g

Good for chewing and swallowing difficulties, constipation (use brown rice), dry mouth, fatigue, mouth and throat sores, and weight gain.

Pacific Steamed Fish

Yield: 2 servings
Preparation time: 5 minutes to assemble; 15 minutes to cook

1 teaspoon sesame oil

1 pound halibut fillets, rinsed and dried

2 well-washed scallions, chopped

1 tablespoon soy sauce

2 tablespoons water

This low-fat dish is mildly spiced to let the flavor of the fish come through.

1. Place the oil in a large frying pan over low heat. Add the fish, and cover with the remaining ingredients.

2. Cover, and cook for 15 minutes, or until the fish flakes easily when tested with a fork. Serve immediately.

NUTRITION INFORMATION (PER SERVING):
Calories: 275   Fat: 7 g   Carbohydrate: 1 g   Protein: 48 g

Good for chewing and swallowing difficulties, fatigue, loss of appetite, and nausea and vomiting.

Modification

If experiencing diarrhea, omit the scallions. The nutrition information doesn't change.

Cornmeal Fish Fillets

Yield: 2 servings
Preparation time: 30 minutes

1 tablespoon lemon or lime juice

2 halibut fillets (6 ounces each), rinsed and dried

¼ cup yellow cornmeal

2 tablespoons grated Parmesan cheese

¼ to ½ teaspoon fennel seeds, crushed (optional)

1 tablespoon olive oil

Feel free to add your favorite spices to the cornmeal mixture, especially if you are experiencing alterations in taste.

1. Place the lemon or lime juice in a shallow bowl, and marinate the fish in the juice for 10 minutes.

2. Place the cornmeal, cheese, and fennel in a small bowl, and mix thoroughly. Dip the fish in this mixture until completely coated.

3. Place the oil in a large frying pan over medium-high heat. Add the fish, and cook about 6 minutes on each side, or until the fish is flaky when tested with a fork. Serve immediately.

NUTRITION INFORMATION (PER SERVING):

Calories: 330   Fat: 14 g   Carbohydrate: 13 g   Protein: 39 g

---

Good for alterations in taste, chewing and swallowing difficulties, loss of appetite, and weight gain.

Modification

If experiencing constipation, omit the regular cornmeal, and use ¼ cup whole grain cornmeal. The nutrition information doesn't change.

Baked Parmesan Fish Fillets

Yield: 2 servings
Preparation time: 15 minutes to assemble; 15 to 20 minutes to bake

¾ cup plain low-fat yogurt

⅓ cup grated Parmesan cheese

2 teaspoons lemon juice

1 small onion, finely minced or grated

¼ teaspoon salt

½ small dried red chili pepper, seeded and crushed

2 firm halibut fillets (5 ounces each), rinsed and dried

1 teaspoon ground paprika

The yogurt in this recipe helps to keep the fish moist and tender.

1. Preheat the oven to 350°F.

2. Place the yogurt, cheese, lemon juice, onion, salt, and chili pepper in a medium-sized bowl, and mix thoroughly.

3. Coat an 8-inch square baking dish with with nonstick cooking spray. Place the fish in the baking dish. Pour the yogurt mixture over the fish, and sprinkle with the paprika. Bake for 15 to 20 minutes, or until the fish flakes easily when tested with a fork. Serve immediately.

NUTRITION INFORMATION (PER SERVING):
Calories: 335   Fat: 10 g   Carbohydrate: 11 g   Protein: 47 g

Good for alterations in taste, chewing and swallowing difficulties, fatigue, and weight gain.

Poached Fish

Yield: 4 servings
Preparation time: 3 minutes to assemble; 7 to 10 minutes to cook

2 cups water

3 tablespoons lemon juice

1 medium-sized onion, sliced

1 bay leaf

2 whole cloves

1 ½ pounds halibut fillets, rinsed and dried

This quick and easy dish can be served hot with lemon juice or cold with a green salad.

1. Place the water, lemon juice, onion, bay leaf, and cloves in a large frying pan over medium heat, and bring to a simmer.

2. Add the fish, cover, and adjust the heat to maintain a simmer. Cook for 7 to 10 minutes, or until fish flakes easily when tested with a fork.

3. Use a spatula to lift the fish from the pan, taking care to not break the fillets. Serve immediately, or chill in the refrigerator before serving.

NUTRITION INFORMATION (PER SERVING):

Calories: 205   Fat: 4 g   Carbohydrate: 2 g   Protein: 33 g

Good for alterations in taste, chewing and swallowing difficulties, loss of appetite, and nausea and vomiting.

Modification

If experiencing diarrhea, omit the onion, and use 2 tablespoons onion powder. The nutrition information doesn't change.

Pineapple Salmon Steaks

Yield: 4 servings
Preparation time: 5 minutes to assemble; 7 to 10 minutes to cook

¼ teaspoon salt

¼ teaspoon black pepper

2 tablespoons lemon juice, preferably fresh-squeezed

4 salmon steaks, rinsed and dried

PINEAPPLE SAUCE

1 can (12 ounces) unsweetened crushed pineapple, drained

1 tablespoon Dijon mustard

Sweet pineapple and tangy mustard combine to form the perfect sauce for salmon.

1. Place the salt, pepper, and lemon juice in a medium-sized bowl. Then place each steak in the bowl, and coat with the seasonings.

2. To make the sauce, place the pineapple in a blender, and purée. Add the mustard, and mix thoroughly. Set aside and keep cold.

3. Grill the fish over coals or under the broiler for about 7 to 10 minutes, or until it flakes when tested with a fork. Serve with the pineapple sauce.

NUTRITION INFORMATION (PER SERVING):

Calories: 240   Fat: 8 g   Carbohydrate: 8 g   Protein: 33 g

Good for alterations in taste, chewing and swallowing difficulties, dry mouth, fatigue, loss of appetite, and nausea and vomiting.

Tuna Bake

Yield: 4 servings
Preparation time: 10 minutes to
assemble; 20 minutes to bake

1 can (6 ounces) water-packed
   tuna, drained

1 can (10 ¾ ounces)
   condensed tomato soup

½ cup low-fat milk

1 cup shredded cheddar cheese

1 pound macaroni, cooked and
   drained (measured before
   cooking)

*Remember Mom's tuna casserole? She really did know what was good for
you. This is our fast and tasty version of a standard comfort food.*

1. Preheat the oven to 350°F.

2. Place tuna, tomato soup, milk, and cheese in large saucepan over
medium heat. Mix thoroughly. Cook until cheese melts, about 10 minutes.

3. Add the macaroni to the sauce, and mix thoroughly.

4. Coat an 8-inch square baking dish with nonstick cooking spray. Pour
the macaroni mixture into the baking dish, and bake, uncovered, for 20
minutes, or until hot and bubbly. Serve immediately.

NUTRITION INFORMATION (PER SERVING):

Calories: 680   Fat: 13 g   Carbohydrate: 100 g   Protein: 37 g

Good for alterations in taste, chewing and swallowing difficulties,
dry mouth, fatigue, and weight gain.

Salmon Loaf

Yield: 6 servings
Preparation time: 10 minutes to
assemble; 45 minutes to bake

2 cans (6 ounces each)
   water-packed salmon,
   drained (reserve liquid)

2 eggs

1 cup low-fat milk

3 cups cracker crumbs

2 tablespoons lemon juice

2 teaspoons chopped onion

¼ teaspoon salt

¼ teaspoon black pepper

Try this dish as a tasty change of pace from your regular meat loaf.

1. Preheat the oven to 350°F.

2. Place the salmon and eggs in a large bowl, and mix thoroughly.

3. Place the milk and ½ cup of the salmon liquid in a small bowl, and
stir. Stir the liquid and the remaining ingredients into the salmon mixture.

4. Coat a loaf pan with nonstick cooking spray. Spoon the salmon
mixture into the loaf pan. Bake, uncovered, for about 45 minutes, or until
thoroughly heated. Serve immediately.

NUTRITION INFORMATION (PER SERVING):

Calories: 355   Fat: 11 g   Carbohydrate: 48 g   Protein: 14 g

Good for alterations in taste, dry mouth, and weight gain.

Modifications

If experiencing chewing and swallowing difficulties, omit the onions, and use $\frac{1}{8}$ teaspoon of onion powder. The nutrition information doesn't change.

If experiencing mouth and throat sores, omit the lemon juice. The nutrition information doesn't change.

Oven Fried Scallops

Yield: 2 servings
Preparation time: 10 minutes to assemble; 12 minutes to bake

1 cup bread crumbs

½ teaspoon salt

¼ teaspoon white pepper

½ teaspoon ground paprika

4 eggs

½ pound large scallops, rinsed and dried

This a great way to prepare these sweet, tender morsels.

1. Preheat the oven to 450°F.

2. Place the bread crumbs, salt, pepper, and paprika in a medium-sized bowl, and mix thoroughly. Place the eggs in another medium-sized bowl, and beat with a fork.

3. Dip each scallop in the egg, and then in the bread crumb mixture. Make sure the scallops are well coated.

4. Coat a cookie sheet with nonstick cooking spray. Place the scallops on the cookie sheet, and bake for about 12 minutes, or until scallops are crisp on the outside and soft on the inside. Serve immediately.

NUTRITION INFORMATION (PER SERVING):

Calories: 225   Fat: 2 g   Carbohydrate: 14 g   Protein: 35 g

Good for diarrhea, loss of appetite, and nausea and vomiting.

Mediterranean Baked Shrimp

Yield: 4 servings
Preparation time: 45 minutes

A must for shrimp lovers. Either have the fish seller devein the shrimp, or do it yourself—see "Deveining Shrimp."

1 tablespoon olive oil

4 large well-washed scallions, minced

1 garlic clove, minced

1 pound large shrimp, peeled and deveined

4 well-washed plum tomatoes, diced

½ cup crumbled feta cheese

2 large eggs

1 tablespoon finely chopped fresh dill, or 1 teaspoon dried

¼ teaspoon hot pepper sauce

¼ teaspoon salt

¼ teaspoon black pepper

½ cup low-fat milk

1 tablespoon grated Parmesan cheese

1. Preheat the oven to 400°F.

2. Place the oil in a small frying pan over medium heat. Add the scallions, and cook, stirring frequently, until softened—about 3 minutes. Add the garlic and cook, stirring, for 1 minute.

3. Coat a 9-inch pie pan or baking dish with nonstick cooking spray. Spread the scallion mixture in the pie pan or baking dish, and arrange the shrimp on top. Sprinkle with the tomatoes and feta cheese.

4. Place the eggs, dill, pepper sauce, salt, and black pepper in a small bowl, and beat together. Beat in the milk.

5. Spoon the egg mixture over shrimp, and sprinkle with the cheese. Bake for 17 minutes, or until the egg mixture is set and the shrimp are cooked thoroughly. Let stand 5 minutes before serving.

NUTRITION INFORMATION (PER SERVING):

Calories: 270   Fat: 15 g   Carbohydrate: 7 g   Protein: 27 g

---

Good for alterations in taste, loss of appetite, and weight gain.

Deveining Shrimp

The vein, the dark cord that runs down the center of the shrimp's back, should be removed. The easiest way to devein shrimp is to have your local fish store do it, especially when you're buying a lot of them. However, if you want to do it yourself, you can do so with either the point of a small knife or a toothpick, as shown.

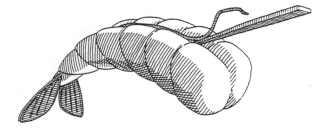

Microwave Easy Crab Delight

Yield: 1 serving
Preparation time: 8 minutes

1 can (5 ounces) crab meat, drained

1 tablespoon wine vinegar

¼ cup shredded mozzarella cheese

Try this tasty crab creation over toast or bread, or tuck it in a pita pocket or tortilla. If you want more texture in your meal, add cut-up carrots or celery after microwaving. For a spicy variation, try adding honey mustard.

1. Place the crab meat in a microwave-safe dish, and sprinkle with the vinegar and cheese.

2. Cover with microwave-safe plastic wrap, and cook on high power for 2 to 3 minutes, or until thoroughly heated. Serve immediately.

NUTRITION INFORMATION (PER SERVING):
Calories: 220   Fat: 8 g   Carbohydrate: 1 g   Protein: 35 g

Good for chewing and swallowing difficulties, dry mouth, fatigue, and weight gain.

Modification

If experiencing mouth and throat sores, omit the vinegar, and use 1 tablespoon low-fat milk.

MODIFIED NUTRITION INFORMATION:
Calories: 225   Fat: 8 g   Carbohydrate: 1 g   Protein: 35 g

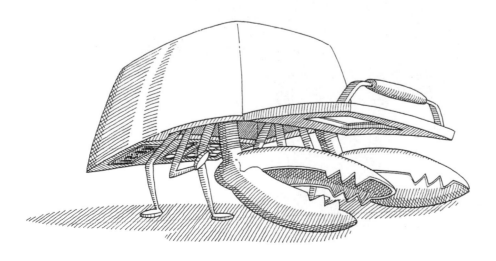

Beef Stroganoff

Yield: 4 servings
Preparation time: 30 minutes

1 tablespoon canola oil

1 garlic clove, minced

⅓ cup chopped onion

1 pound extra-lean ground beef

2 tablespoons white flour

1 teaspoon salt

1 teaspoon ground paprika

2 cans (3 ounces each) sliced
   mushrooms

1 can (10 ¾ ounces)
   condensed cream of chicken
   soup

1 cup plain low-fat yogurt

½ pound wide, flat noodles,
   cooked and drained
   (measured before cooking)

2 tablespoons chopped
   well-washed parsley

This traditional dish is very filling.

1. Place the oil in a frying pan over medium heat. Add the garlic, onion, and beef, and cook until the meat is no longer pink, about 8 to 10 minutes. Drain off any fat.

2. Add the flour, salt, paprika, and mushrooms, and stir. Add the soup, reduce the heat to low, and simmer for 10 minutes.

3. Stir in the yogurt, keeping the heat low, and let the mixture heat through. Serve over the noodles, and sprinkle with the parsley.

NUTRITION INFORMATION (PER SERVING):

Calories: 600   Fat: 25 g   Carbohydrate: 57 g   Protein: 36 g

---

Good for chewing and swallowing difficulties, dry mouth, mouth and throat sores, and weight gain.

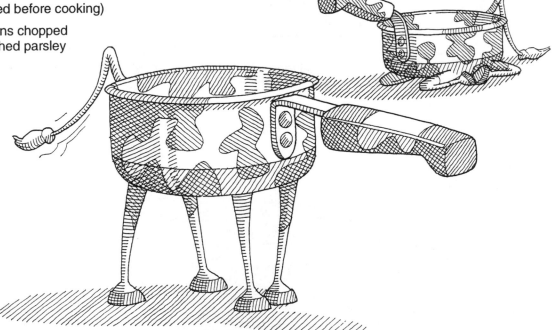

Hometown Burgers

Yield: 4 servings
Preparation time: 20 to 40 minutes, depending on cooking method

1 pound extra-lean ground beef

1 egg, beaten

½ cup bread crumbs

¼ cup ketchup

1 teaspoon Worcestershire sauce

1 teaspoon salt

1 teaspoon black pepper

1 teaspoon garlic powder

Dress up this basic burger with your favorite condiments and vegetable toppings. Try grilled tomato or mushrooms, cheese slices, sweet onions, guacamole, or Thousand Island dressing.

1. Place all of the ingredients in a large bowl, and mix thoroughly. Form into 4 patties.

2. Broil or grill the patties until the meat is cooked all the way through, about 7 to 10 minutes a side. Or, bake at 350°F for 35 minutes. Serve on hamburger buns or bread.

NUTRITION INFORMATION (PER SERVING):

Calories: 380   Fat: 17 g   Carbohydrate: 28 g   Protein: 27 g

---

Good for alterations in taste, chewing and swallowing difficulties (use soft bread), and weight gain.

Mini Meat Loaves

Yield: 4 servings
Preparation time: 15 minutes to assemble; 25 to 30 minutes to bake

1 pound extra-lean ground beef

¾ cup uncooked rolled oats

½ cup finely chopped onion

1 teaspoon baking powder

Try this recipe with ground turkey if you crave a change.

1. Preheat the oven to 375°F.

2. Place all of the ingredients in a large bowl, and mix thoroughly. Form into four loaves about 2 inches high.

3. Place the loaves in a large, ungreased baking dish, and bake until brown and cooked through, about 25 to 30 minutes. Serve immediately.

NUTRITION INFORMATION (PER SERVING):

Calories: 275   Fat: 13 g   Carbohydrate: 12 g   Protein: 20 g

---

Good for chewing and swallowing difficulties, constipation, dry mouth, fatigue, loss of appetite, and mouth and throat sores.

Hamburger Noodle Feast

Yield: 6 servings
Preparation time: 20 minutes to assemble; 30 minutes to bake

1 pound uncooked noodles

1 pound extra-lean ground beef

2 large onions, chopped

1 jar (24 ounces) spaghetti sauce

1 cup sliced well-washed mushrooms

1 package (10 ounces) frozen corn kernels, unthawed

1 package (10 ounces) frozen peas, unthawed

1 cup shredded cheddar cheese

This casserole is hearty and satisfying.

1. Preheat the oven to 350°F.

2. Cook the noodles according to the package directions, but remove from the heat and drain when they are slightly underdone.

3. Place the beef and onions in a large nonstick frying pan over medium-high heat, and cook until the meat is no longer pink, about 10 minutes. Drain any fat. Add the spaghetti sauce, and simmer for a few minutes.

4. Place the meat mixture in a 9-x-13-inch baking dish, and add the noodles, mushrooms, corn, and peas. Mix thoroughly. Top with the cheese, cover, and bake for 30 minutes, or until hot and bubbly. Serve immediately.

NUTRITION INFORMATION (PER SERVING):

Calories: 645   Fat: 20 g   Carbohydrate: 81 g   Protein: 36 g

---

Good for alterations in taste, constipation, dry mouth, and weight gain.

Oven Meatballs

Yield: 6 servings
Preparation time: 15 minutes to assemble; 30 minutes to bake

1 cup bread crumbs

4 egg whites

½ cup water

1 teaspoon ketchup

1 teaspoon onion powder

1 teaspoon salt

1 teaspoon black pepper

1 teaspoon ground paprika

1 ½ pounds extra-lean ground beef

Serve these meatballs over your favorite pasta with tomato sauce.

1. Preheat the oven to 350°F.

2. Place the bread crumbs in a large bowl. Add the egg whites and water, and blend slightly with a fork. Add the ketchup, onion powder, salt, pepper, and paprika. Add the beef, and mix thoroughly.

3. Roll the meat mixture into 2-inch balls, and place in a 9-x-13-inch baking dish. Bake for 30 minutes, or until the meatballs are no longer pink inside.

NUTRITION INFORMATION (PER SERVING):

Calories: 240   Fat: 10 g   Carbohydrate: 5 g   Protein: 29 g

---

Good for chewing and swallowing difficulties, diarrhea, dry mouth, loss of appetite, mouth and throat sores, and nausea and vomiting.

Tamale Pie

Yield: 4 servings
Preparation time: 40 minutes

1 pound extra-lean ground beef

2 cans (15 ounces each) creamed corn

¾ cup cornmeal

1 can (15 ounces) tomato sauce

1 teaspoon dry taco seasoning

1 can (4 ounces) sliced olives

Top this pie with cheese, plain low-fat yogurt, or guacamole.

1. Preheat the oven to 400°F.

2. Place the beef in a large nonstick frying pan, and cook until no longer pink, about 8 to 10 minutes. Drain off any fat. Add the remaining ingredients, and mix thoroughly.

3. Coat a 9-x-13-inch baking dish with nonstick cooking spray. Pour the meat mixture into the dish, and bake for 30 minutes, or until thoroughly heated. Serve immediately.

NUTRITION INFORMATION (PER SERVING):

Calories: 485   Fat: 16 g   Carbohydrate: 64 g   Protein: 28 g

---

Good for alterations in taste, constipation, fatigue, and weight gain.

Sloppy Joes

Yield: 2 servings
Preparation time: 30 minutes

½ pound extra-lean ground beef

1 small onion, diced

½ cup prepared barbecue sauce

1 tablespoon uncooked rolled oats

Water

This is another classic dish that's good, and good for you.

1. Place the beef and onion in a small frying pan over medium-high heat. Cook until the meat is no longer pink, about 8 to 10 minutes. Pour off any fat.

2. Add the barbecue sauce and oats, and enough water to cover the meat. Bring to a boil, then turn down the heat until the mixture simmers. Cover, and cook 15 minutes, or until the sauce has thickened and the meat is soft. Serve on buns, toast, or hard rolls.

NUTRITION INFORMATION (PER SERVING):

Calories: 410   Fat: 17 g   Carbohydrate: 35 g   Protein: 27 g

---

Good for alterations in taste, chewing and swallowing difficulties, dry mouth (use soft bread), fatigue, and weight gain.

Modification

If experiencing diarrhea or nausea and vomiting, omit the beef and use ½ pound extra-lean ground turkey. Use a mild barbecue sauce. Omit the onions, and use 1 tablespoon onion powder.

MODIFIED NUTRITION INFORMATION:

Calories: 330   Fat: 10 g   Carbohydrate: 34 g   Protein: 20 g

---

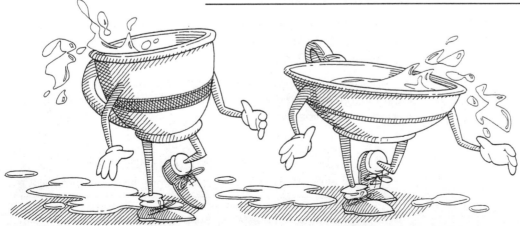

Pork Chop Baked With Apples and Sweet Potatoes

Yield: 1 serving
Preparation time: 15 minutes to assemble; 40 minutes to bake

1 lean pork chop

1 medium-sized, well-washed sweet potato, peeled and thinly sliced

1 small, well-washed apple, cored and sliced

1 tablespoon raisins

1 teaspoon ground cinnamon

Having trouble deciding what to cook for one? Here's a simple and flavorful answer.

1. Preheat the oven to 350°F.

2. Place the pork chop, sweet potato, and apple on a large piece of foil. Top with the raisins and cinnamon.

3. Wrap well, and bake for 40 minutes, or until the chop is cooked through. Serve immediately.

NUTRITION INFORMATION (PER SERVING):

Calories: 465   Fat: 16 g   Carbohydrate: 57 g   Protein: 26 g

---

Good for fatigue, loss of appetite, and nausea and vomiting.

Sweet and Spicy Pork Chops

Yield: 4 servings
Preparation time: 15 minutes to assemble; 45 minutes to bake

1 tablespoon canola oil

4 pork chops, trimmed of fat

¼ cup apricot preserves

¼ cup pineapple preserves

¼ cup soy sauce

¼ cup wine vinegar

The preserves not only make this dish sweet, but also help to keep the meat moist.

1. Preheat the oven to 350°F.

2. Place the oil in a large frying pan over medium-high heat. Add the chops, and cook until brown on both sides, about 2 minutes a side. Place the chops in a 9-x-13-inch baking dish.

3. Place the remaining ingredients in a medium-sized bowl, and mix thoroughly. Pour over the chops, cover, and bake for 45 minutes, or until the chops are cooked all the way through. Serve immediately.

NUTRITION INFORMATION (PER SERVING):

Calories: 300   Fat: 11 g   Carbohydrate: 30 g   Protein: 19 g

---

Good for alterations in taste, fatigue, and loss of appetite.

Vegetarian Entrées

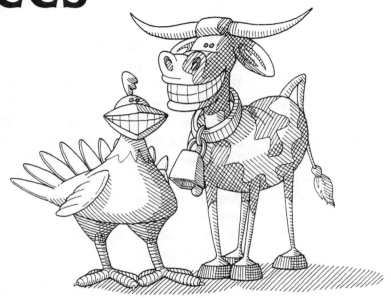

Vegetarianism may appeal to someone with HIV for many reasons, including an inability to chew and swallow meats. Also, a distaste for meat may occur as a side effect of medication. Even if you are not a strict vegetarian, you will find these entrées thoroughly pleasing.

The recipes in this chapter are primarily lacto-ovo vegetarian dishes, meaning that many of them contain dairy and eggs. These recipes are designed to help you meet your protein requirements without the addition of meat. See page 212 for instructions on cooking dry legumes, page 213 for instructions on cooking rice, and page 178 for instructions on cooking vegetables.

Vegans, or vegetarians who eat no dairy foods or eggs, need to include plenty of calcium-rich nondairy foods in their diet. These include legumes, soybeans, almonds, tahini, kale, bok choy, mustard greens, broccoli, corn tortillas, and seaweed.

If you have trouble gaining or maintaining weight on a vegetarian diet, eat more high-calorie vegetarian foods, such as nuts, legumes, grains, and dairy products. If you're considering switching to a vegetarian diet, consult a registered dietitian to help you get started on meal plans that will provide you with the nutrients your body requires.

Recipe-By-Symptoms Chart

Different recipes in this section are designed to address different symptoms that commonly occur in people with HIV disease. This chart can help you find recipes to ease your symptoms. You'll note that some recipes address multiple symptoms.

ALTERATIONS IN TASTE	Bean and Cheese Enchiladas, Bean Stew With Couscous, Greek Pasta, India Casserole, Nutty Noodles, Panama Pasta, Tofu Egg Salad Sandwich, Vegetarian Sloppy Joes
CHEWING AND SWALLOWING DIFFICULTIES	Bean Stew With Couscous, India Casserole (modified), Italian Bulgur Bake (modified), Macaroni and Cheese, Panama Pasta, Traditional Egg Salad Sandwich
CONSTIPATION	Bean and Cheese Enchiladas, Bean Stew With Couscous, Cheesy Bean and Rice Casserole, Cheesy Pasta Primavera, Double Nut Sandwich, India Casserole, Microwave Lentil Burritos, Tofu Rice Burgers
DIARRHEA	Tofu Egg Salad Sandwich, Tofu Rice Burgers (modified), Vegetarian Sloppy Joes
DRY MOUTH	Bean Stew With Couscous, Italian Bulgur Bake, Macaroni and Cheese, Panama Pasta, Traditional Egg Salad Sandwich, Vegetarian Sloppy Joes
FATIGUE	Bean and Cheese Enchiladas, Cheesy Bean and Rice Casserole, Cheesy Pasta Primavera, Double Nut Sandwich, Greek Pasta, India Casserole, Italian Bulgur Bake, Microwave Lentil Burritos, Nutty Noodles, Traditional Egg Salad Sandwich, Vegetarian Sloppy Joes
LOSS OF APPETITE	Bean and Cheese Enchiladas, Cheesy Bean and Rice Casserole, Double Nut Sandwich, Greek Pasta, India Casserole, Microwave Lentil Burritos, Panama Pasta, Traditional Egg Salad Sandwich, Vegetarian Sloppy Joes
MOUTH AND THROAT SORES	Cheesy Pasta Primavera, Macaroni and Cheese, Traditional Egg Salad Sandwich (modified)

NAUSEA AND VOMITING	Bean Stew With Couscous, Cheesy Pasta Primavera, Tofu Egg Salad Sandwich, Tofu Rice Burgers (modified)
WEIGHT GAIN	Bean and Cheese Enchiladas, Bean Stew With Couscous, Cheesy Bean and Rice Casserole, Cheesy Pasta Primavera, Double Nut Sandwich, Greek Pasta, India Casserole, Italian Bulgur Bake, Macaroni and Cheese, Microwave Lentil Burritos, Nutty Noodles, Panama Pasta, Tofu Rice Burgers, Traditional Egg Salad Sandwich

Bean and Cheese Enchiladas

*Yield: 6 enchiladas
Preparation time: 20 minutes
to assemble; 30 to 35 minutes
to bake*

1 ½ cups refried beans

1 ½ cups low-fat cottage
cheese

¾ cup chopped onion

2 cups enchilada sauce,
canned or homemade

6 corn tortillas

HOMEMADE ENCHILADA SAUCE

½ cup tomato sauce

1 teaspoon chili powder

¼ teaspoon garlic powder

1 ½ teaspoons onion powder

¼ teaspoon black pepper

⅛ teaspoon cayenne pepper

1 ½ cups plus 1 tablespoon
water, divided

1 ½ teaspoons cornstarch

If you've found a brand of canned enchilada sauce that you like, fine. But why not try ours? If you like our homemade sauce, you can easily double the ingredients and freeze the leftovers for up to 3 months. This recipe is quick and easy to prepare.

1. Preheat the oven to 450°F.

2. Place the beans, cheese, and onion in a medium-sized bowl, and mix thoroughly. Set aside.

3. To make the the sauce, place the first six ingredients and 1 ½ cups of the water in a large saucepan over medium heat, and cook until the mixture comes to a boil. Then reduce the heat to low, and simmer for 10 minutes. After the sauce simmers, place the remaining 1 tablespoon of water in a cup, and dissolve the cornstarch in it. Add the cornstarch mixture to the sauce, a little at a time, stirring constantly until the sauce thickens.

4. Coat a 9-inch square baking dish with nonstick cooking spray. Pour one cup of the sauce into the dish, and spread it evenly over the bottom.

5. Steam the tortillas for a few minutes, or place in a microwave-safe plastic bag and microwave on high power for 10 seconds.

6. Divide the bean mixture into 6 even portions. Place a portion on each of the tortillas, and spread into an even layer. Then roll up each tortilla and place, seam side down, in the baking dish.

7. Pour the remaining sauce over the enchiladas. Bake 30 to 35 minutes, or until the top is crisp, the sauce is bubbly, and the cheese begins to melt. Serve immediately.

NUTRITION INFORMATION (PER 2-ENCHILADA SERVING):
Calories: 415   Fat: 6 g   Carbohydrate: 61 g   Protein: 28 g

Good for alterations in taste, constipation, fatigue (use canned sauce),
loss of appetite, and weight gain.

Bean Stew With Couscous

Yield: 6 servings
Preparation time: 50 minutes

¼ cup canola oil

1 large onion, finely chopped

1 large, well-washed green bell pepper, seeded and chopped

1 large, well-washed red bell pepper, seeded and chopped

1 teaspoon ground coriander

1 teaspoon ground cinnamon

2 medium-sized, well-washed sweet potatoes, peeled and cut into ½-inch cubes

2 large, well-washed tomatoes, chopped

1 tablespoon lemon juice

2 cups garbanzo beans, cooked fresh or canned, rinsed and drained

1 teaspoon salt

1 medium-sized, well-washed zucchini, chopped

4 ¼ cups water, divided

2 cups uncooked couscous

Couscous, a crumb-like pasta, is a staple in North Africa. Look for couscous in your favorite health food store or supermarket. If you're using dry garbanzo beans, see page 212 for cooking instructions.

1. Place the oil in a 5-quart saucepan over medium heat. Add the onion, green and red peppers, coriander, and cinnamon, and cook, stirring occasionally, until the onion is soft—about 5 minutes. Add the sweet potatoes, stir, and cook for 2 more minutes.

2. Add the tomatoes, lemon juice, garbanzo beans, salt, zucchini, and ¼ cup of the water. Cover, reduce the heat, and simmer for 15 minutes.

3. While the stew is simmering, mix the couscous with the remaining water in a medium-sized saucepan over medium-high heat. Bring to a boil, then turn off the heat and let stand for 5 minutes, or until soft.

4. To serve, spread the couscous around the edge of a plate, and spoon the stew into the center. Top with hot pepper sauce, if desired.

NUTRITION INFORMATION (PER SERVING):

Calories: 355   Fat: 10 g   Carbohydrate: 57 g   Protein: 11 g

---

Good for alterations in taste, chewing and swallowing difficulties, constipation, dry mouth, nausea and vomiting, and weight gain.

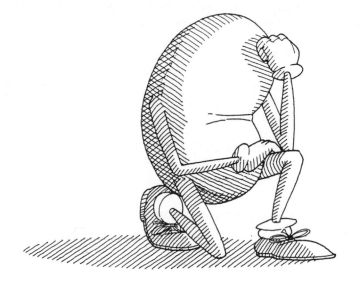

Cheesy Bean and Rice Casserole

Yield: 6 servings
Preparation time: 15 minutes to assemble; 30 minutes to bake

3 cups cooked brown rice

2 cans (16 ounces each) kidney beans, rinsed and drained

1 large onion, chopped

1 teaspoon garlic powder

1 cup low-fat cottage cheese

1 tablespoon white flour

1 can (4 ounces) green chili peppers, diced

2 medium-sized, well-washed tomatoes, chopped, or 1 can (16 ounces) stewed tomatoes

1 ½ cups shredded cheddar or hot pepper jack cheese

Feel free to use your favorite cheese in this dish. To spice it up, use hot pepper jack. If you prefer a milder dish, try cheddar. See "Cooking Rice."

1. Preheat the oven to 350°F.

2. Place the rice, beans, onion, garlic, cottage cheese, flour, and chili peppers in a large bowl, and mix thoroughly.

3. Pour the mixture into a 9-x-13-inch baking dish. Pour the tomatoes over the top, and then add the shredded cheese.

4. Cover, and bake for 30 minutes, or until thoroughly heated. Serve immediately.

NUTRITION INFORMATION (PER SERVING):

Calories: 370   Fat: 12 g   Carbohydrate: 46 g   Protein: 21 g

---

Good for constipation, fatigue, loss of appetite, and weight gain.

Cooking Dry Beans and Peas

Dried beans and peas are known as legumes. They are highly nutritious, low in fat, and inexpensive, and they have more protein than any other vegetable food. Legumes are, however, an incomplete protein (see page 8), so you will need to serve them with a complementary grain-based protein. Try legumes in stews, casseroles, salads, and soups.

To cook dry beans and peas:

1. Sort through the dry beans, and discard any that are discolored or shriveled. Rinse well. Drain.

2. Soak the beans, except for lentils. This softens them, resulting in faster cooking time. It helps to reduce the intestinal gas some people experience after eating beans—and the more often you eat beans, the less problems you'll have. There are two ways of soaking beans:

Quick Soak: Place 1 pound of beans and 6 cups of water in a pot over high heat, and bring to a boil. Boil for 2 minutes. Remove the pot from the heat and let it stand, covered, for 1 hour. Drain and rinse well.

Overnight Soak: Place 1 pound of beans or peas in 6 cups of water in a large bowl, and soak overnight. The beans will swell as they soak, so use a larger bowl than you think you'll need! Drain and rinse well.

3. Place the beans and fresh water to cover in a pot over high heat, and bring to a boil. Reduce heat to low, cover, and simmer until tender. Stir occasionally. To reduce gas after eating, change water at least once during the cooking process, being careful to bring the beans back to a simmer. Most varieties take 1½ to 2 hours to cook. Soybeans may take 3 hours.

Cooking Rice

If the only rice you've ever eaten is white rice, you might want to try brown rice for a flavorful change of pace. Brown rice has had only the inedible outer hull removed, while white rice has had both the hull and the middle bran layer removed. This means that brown rice is more nutritious, since fewer nutrients are lost during processing. However, brown rice does take longer to cook. Rice also varies in the length of the grains: short, medium, and long.

There are also specialty rices, such as wild rice and the aromatic Basmati rice. Converted or parboiled rice is soaked and steamed under pressure before the bran is removed. This leaves the rice with more of its original nutrients, and with a fluffier texture.

Different types of rice require different amounts of liquid and cooking times:

Per 1 cup uncooked	Liquid	Cooking Time	Serving
Long-grain white	2 cups	20 minutes	3 $\frac{1}{2}$ cups
Medium- or short-grain white	1 $\frac{1}{2}$ cup	20 minutes	3 $\frac{1}{2}$ cups
Long-grain brown	2 cups	25 to 35 minutes	3 cups
Short-grain brown	2 cups	40 minutes	3 cups
Wild	4 cups	50 minutes	4 cups
Parboiled/converted	2 $\frac{2}{3}$ cups	30 to 35 minutes	4 cups

You can cook rice either on the stovetop or in the microwave:

Stovetop: Place the rice, liquid, 1 teaspoon salt (optional), and 1 tablespoon butter (optional) in a 2- to 3-quart saucepan over high heat. Bring to a boil, stirring once or twice. Then lower the heat to a simmer, cover with a tight-fitting lid, and cook for the time shown on the chart. If the rice is not tender or the liquid is not absorbed at the end of that time, replace the lid and cook 2 to 4 more minutes.

Microwave: Place the rice, liquid, 1 teaspoon salt (optional), and 1 tablespoon butter (optional) in a 2- to 3-quart deep, microwave-safe baking dish. Cover, and cook on high for 5 minutes, or until the liquid is boiling. Then reduce the power to medium, and cook 15 minutes for white rice, 35 to 45 minutes for brown rice, 20 to 30 minutes for wild rice, and 15 to 22 minutes for parboiled/converted rice. Cook until the liquid is absorbed and the rice is tender. After cooking, let stand, covered, for 5 minutes.

Italian Bulgur Bake

Yield: 4 servings
Preparation time: 1 hour

2 cups canned kidney beans, rinsed and drained

1 can (16 ounces) whole tomatoes, drained and diced

1 medium-sized, well-washed zucchini, halved lengthwise and sliced

½ cup uncooked bulgur

½ cup chopped onion

½ teaspoon salt

½ teaspoon dried oregano, or 1 teaspoon chopped fresh

¼ teaspoon black pepper

¾ cup shredded mozzarella cheese

You can also make this dish with leftover beef, pork, or lamb—just use the meat in place of the beans. See page 168 for information on bulgur.

1. Preheat the oven to 375°F.

2. Place all the ingredients except the cheese in a 8-inch square baking dish, and mix thoroughly.

3. Bake, covered, for 45 to 50 minutes, or until heated through. Sprinkle with the cheese, and bake, uncovered, for an additional 5 minutes, or until the cheese melts. Serve immediately.

NUTRITION INFORMATION (PER SERVING):

Calories: 340   Fat: 12 g   Carbohydrate: 42 g   Protein: 20 g

---

Good for dry mouth, fatigue, and weight gain.

Modification

If experiencing chewing and swallowing difficulties, omit the onion, and use 1 teaspoon onion powder. The nutrition information doesn't change.

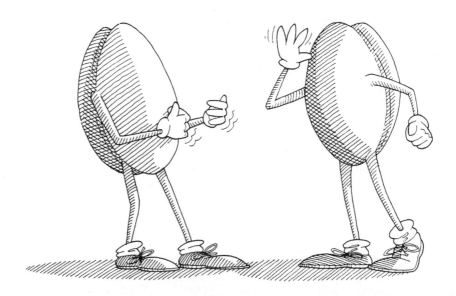

Cheesy Pasta Primavera

Yield: 4 servings
Preparation time: 35 minutes

½ pound cooked pasta
  (measured before cooking)

1 cup ricotta cheese

4 cups steamed, cut-up
  well-washed vegetables,
  such as broccoli,
  mushrooms, carrots, squash,
  or spinach

2 teaspoons seasoning, such
  as dried oregano or basil (or
  ¼ cup fresh), garlic powder,
  chopped fresh parsley, or
  Parmesan cheese

Vary your vegetables according to your symptoms and tolerances. To reduce the preparation time, use chopped, frozen vegetables cooked according to package directions. If you're not sure how to steam vegetables, see page 178.

1. Place all the ingredients in a large bowl, and toss together. Serve immediately.

NUTRITION INFORMATION (PER SERVING):
Calories: 335   Fat: 6 g   Carbohydrate: 54 g   Protein: 16 g

---

Good for constipation, fatigue, mouth and throat sores,
nausea and vomiting, and weight gain.

Macaroni and Cheese

Yield: 2 servings
Preparation time: 20 minutes to
assemble; 15 minutes to bake

1 cup low-fat milk

1 tablespoon white flour

1 tablespoon butter

1 teaspoon minced onion

1 teaspoon salt

1 teaspoon black pepper

1 teaspoon dry mustard

2 cups cooked elbow macaroni
  (measured before cooking)

1 cup shredded cheddar cheese

This dish may be frozen before baking and kept for up to 3 months if wrapped airtight.

1. Preheat the oven to 400°F.

2. Place the milk, flour, butter, onion, salt, pepper, and dry mustard in a medium-sized saucepan over medium heat, and cook until the mixture thickens. Stir in the macaroni and cheese.

3. Coat an 8-inch square baking dish with nonstick cooking spray. Pour the mixture into the dish and bake, uncovered, for 15 minutes, or until slightly browned and bubbly. Let stand 5 minutes before serving.

NUTRITION INFORMATION (PER SERVING):
Calories: 545   Fat: 26 g   Carbohydrate: 52 g   Protein: 26 g

---

Good for chewing and swallowing difficulties, dry mouth,
mouth and throat sores, and weight gain.

Greek Pasta

Yield: 4 servings
Preparation time: 25 to 28 minutes

4 cups chopped well-washed tomato (about 8 or 9 medium-sized tomatoes)

1 tablespoon olive oil

1 tablespoon red wine vinegar

2 tablespoons chopped well-washed basil

¼ teaspoon salt

¼ teaspoon dried red pepper

1 clove garlic, minced

½ pound cooked angel hair pasta (measured before cooking)

1 cup crumbled feta cheese

Most people think of Italy when they think of pasta, but pasta is also used in Greek cuisine.

1. Place the tomato, oil, vinegar, basil, salt, pepper, and garlic in a medium-sized bowl, and mix thoroughly. Add the pasta and feta cheese, and toss. Serve warm or chilled.

NUTRITION INFORMATION (PER SERVING):
Calories: 560   Fat: 27 g   Carbohydrate: 60 g   Protein: 22 g

---

Good for alterations in taste, fatigue,
loss of appetite, and weight gain.

Double Nut Sandwich

Yield: 1 sandwich
Preparation time: 5 minutes

2 tablespoons peanut butter

2 slices whole grain bread

1 ripe banana, sliced

2 tablespoons granola or sunflower seeds

This sandwich is easy to make and eat anytime—it makes a high-energy meal at school, work, or play. It's also tasty if you toast the bread first, so that the peanut butter melts. Be creative and add flavorings of your choice, such as jam, honey, raisins, maple syrup, or chocolate chips.

1. Spread the peanut butter on the bread, arrange the sliced banana on top of the peanut butter, and sprinkle with the granola or seeds.

NUTRITION INFORMATION (PER SANDWICH):
Calories: 510   Fat: 27 g   Carbohydrate: 60 g   Protein: 17 g

---

Good for constipation, fatigue, loss of appetite, and weight gain.

Panama Pasta

Yield: 8 servings
Preparation time: 50 minutes

1 tablespoon olive oil

1 clove garlic, minced

½ medium-sized onion, chopped

1 medium-sized, well-washed green bell pepper, seeded and chopped

½ cup sliced well-washed mushrooms

1 jar (4 ounces) sun-dried tomatoes in oil, rinsed and drained

1 jar (7 ounces) roasted red peppers

1 jar (14 ounces) spaghetti sauce with tomato and basil

1 teaspoon hot sauce

1 pound uncooked tube-shaped pasta

1 ½ cups shredded mozzarella cheese

You and your friends will soon become addicted to this dish, as is its creator, Matthew. This dish makes great leftovers because the flavors continue to blend after cooking. It is just as good chilled as warm. Serve with a baguette and salad.

1. Preheat the oven to 250°F.

2. Place the oil in a medium-sized saucepan over medium-high heat. Add the garlic, onion, bell pepper, and mushrooms, and sauté until tender-crisp, about 5 minutes.

3. Add the sun-dried tomatoes, roasted peppers, spaghetti sauce, and hot sauce. Let the mixture simmer, uncovered, about 15 minutes.

4. While the sauce simmers, cook the pasta according to the package directions, and drain.

5. Place a third of the pasta in a pasta bowl or 9-x-13-inch baking dish, then top with a third of the sauce and a third of the cheese. Make two more layers. Bake until the cheese melts, about 15 minutes. Serve warm or chilled.

NUTRITION INFORMATION (PER SERVING):

Calories: 530   Fat: 15 g   Carbohydrate: 80 g   Protein: 23 g

Good for alterations in taste, chewing and swallowing difficulties, dry mouth, loss of appetite, and weight gain.

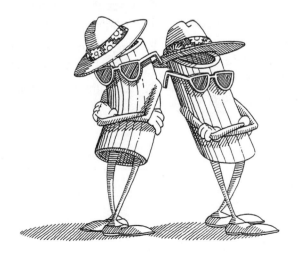

Nutty Noodles

Yield: 4 servings
Preparation time: 25 minutes

⅓ cup peanut butter

1 cup crumbled firm tofu, drained

3 tablespoons soy sauce

3 tablespoons vinegar

1 tablespoon sugar

½ teaspoon dried red pepper, optional

½ pound cooked pasta (measured before cooking)

½ cup nuts, such as peanuts, chopped walnuts, or pine nuts

Our testers could not stop eating these noodles, and they never imagined how versatile peanut butter could be.

1. Place the peanut butter, tofu, soy sauce, vinegar, sugar, and pepper in a small saucepan over medium heat, and cook until the peanut butter is melted and the mixture is heated thoroughly—about 3 minutes.

2. Place the sauce, pasta, and nuts in a large bowl, and toss. Serve warm or chilled.

NUTRITION INFORMATION (PER SERVING):
Calories: 550   Fat: 26 g   Carbohydrate: 58 g   Protein: 28 g

Good for alterations in taste, fatigue, and weight gain.

Vegetarian Sloppy Joes

Yield: 3 servings
Preparation time: 15 minutes to prepare, 1 hour to chill

1 bottle (12 ounces) barbecue or chili sauce

1 pound firm low-fat tofu, drained and crumbled

3 English muffins, split in half

This is not your traditional sloppy joe, but it's just as tasty and easy to make. Cheese makes a nice addition when sprinkled on top.

1. Place the barbecue sauce and tofu in a medium-sized bowl, and mix thoroughly. Cover, and chill for 1 hour.

2. Place the tofu mixture in a large saucepan over medium heat, and cook until hot, about 5 minutes.

3. Toast the English muffins, and top with the tofu mixture.

NUTRITION INFORMATION (PER SERVING):
Calories: 385   Fat: 8 g   Carbohydrate: 53 g   Protein: 28 g

Good for alterations in taste, diarrhea, dry mouth, fatigue, and loss of appetite.

Tofu Egg Salad Sandwich

Yield: 4 sandwiches
Preparation time: 30 minutes

9 eggs

½ cup pickle relish

½ cup crumbled light tofu, drained

1 tablespoon vinegar

1 teaspoon prepared mustard

½ tablespoon salt

If a sandwich doesn't suit you, then simply eat this salad with a spoon or on crackers. Store the unused portion in an airtight container in the refrigerator for up to 2 days.

1. Carefully place the eggs in a large saucepan, and cover with water to two inches above the eggs. Bring the water to a boil. Then cover, turn off the heat, and let sit for 20 minutes. When cooked, run cold water over the eggs, and peel.

2. Place 6 whole eggs and 3 egg whites (discarding 3 yolks) in a large bowl, and chop finely.

3. Add the relish, tofu, vinegar, mustard, and salt to the eggs, and mix thoroughly. Divide evenly to make 4 sandwiches, using white or sourdough bread.

NUTRITION INFORMATION (PER SERVING):
Calories: 325   Fat: 12 g   Carbohydrate: 31 g   Protein: 20 g

---

Good for alterations in taste, diarrhea, and nausea and vomiting.

Microwave Lentil Burritos

Yield: 4 burritos
Preparation time: 7 to 10 minutes

2 ½ cups cooked lentils

1 cup cooked brown rice

¾ cup shredded cheddar cheese

4 flour tortillas

¼ cup prepared salsa

½ cup shredded well-washed lettuce

If you don't have any leftover rice on hand, use instant brown rice and cook according to the package directions. You can also use any type of grain, such as couscous, barley, or bulgur, to suit your taste and tolerances—see page 168 for more information on barley and bulgur. See page 212 for lentil-cooking instructions, or see the microwave directions.

1. Place the lentils, rice, and cheese in a large bowl, and mix thoroughly. Divide evenly among the 4 tortillas.

2. Place each tortilla, open faced, on a microwave-safe plate, and cook each of them for 2 to 5 minutes, or until the cheese is melted.

3. Top with the salsa and lettuce, and then roll into a burrito. Serve immediately.

NUTRITION INFORMATION (PER BURRITO):
Calories: 380   Fat: 10 g   Carbohydrate: 55 g   Protein: 20 g

---

Good for constipation, fatigue, loss of appetite, and weight gain.

Microwave Cooking

To microwave the lentils, combine 1 pound of lentils with 6 cups of water in a microwave-safe dish. Cover, and cook on high power for 10 minutes. Then reduce the power to medium, and cook for an additional 30 to 45 minutes, or until tender. Let stand, still covered, for 10 minutes.

Traditional Egg Salad Sandwich

Yield: 2 sandwiches
Preparation time: 30 minutes

6 eggs
¼ cup pickle relish
¼ cup mayonnaise
4 slices whole wheat bread

If mayonnaise is too rich for you, try substituting plain low-fat yogurt or mashed tofu. You can serve this salad on crackers, or simply eat it with a spoon.

1. Carefully place the eggs in a large saucepan, and cover with water to 2 inches above the eggs. Bring the water to a boil, then cover, turn off the heat, and let sit for 20 minutes. Run cold water over the eggs, and peel.

2. Place the eggs in a medium-sized bowl, and chop finely. Add the pickle relish and mayonnaise to the eggs, and mix thoroughly. Serve on the bread.

NUTRITION INFORMATION (PER SANDWICH):
Calories: 645   Fat: 40 g   Carbohydrate: 45 g   Protein: 26 g

---

Good for chewing and swallowing difficulties, dry mouth (use soft bread), fatigue, loss of appetite, and weight gain.

Modification

If experiencing mouth and throat sores, omit the pickle relish. The nutrition information doesn't change.

India Casserole

Yield: 2 servings
Preparation time: 15 minutes to assemble; 25 to 30 minutes to bake

2 cups cooked brown rice

1 package (10 ounces) frozen peas, thawed and drained

1 ½ cups plain low-fat yogurt

1 cup diced well-washed celery

¼ cup chopped onion

¼ cup chopped nuts, such as peanuts, walnuts, or almonds

¼ cup raisins

1 teaspoon curry powder

2 teaspoons soy sauce

½ teaspoon dry mustard

2 tablespoons grated Parmesan cheese

1 egg white, lightly beaten

This is a great dish to make when you have leftover rice. If you're making rice from scratch, see page 213.

1. Preheat the oven to 350°F.

2. Place all the ingredients in a large bowl, and mix thoroughly.

3. Coat a 9-x-13-inch baking dish with nonstick cooking spray. Pour the mixture into the dish, and bake 25 to 30 minutes, or until heated through. Serve immediately.

NUTRITION INFORMATION (PER SERVING):

Calories: 650   Fat: 16 g   Carbohydrate: 100 g   Protein: 31 g

---

Good for alterations in taste, constipation, loss of appetite, and weight gain. If fatigued, make the dish when feeling well, cover tightly with foil, and freeze for up to 3 months. Adjust the baking time to 1 hour.

Modification

If experiencing chewing and swallowing difficulties, omit the nuts and raisins.

MODIFIED NUTRITION INFORMATION:

Calories: 500   Fat: 7 g   Carbohydrate: 83 g   Protein: 26 g

---

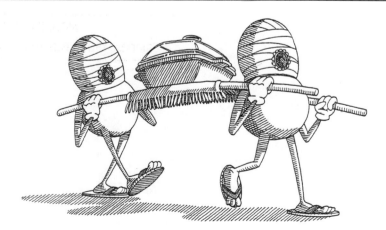

Tofu Rice Burgers

Yield: 4 servings
Preparation time: 15 minutes to assemble; 35 minutes to bake

1 ½ cups crumbled firm light tofu, drained

1 cup cooked brown rice

2 tablespoons chopped onion

2 eggs, lightly beaten

1 teaspoon salt

1 cup bread crumbs

1 teaspoon ground paprika

2 tablespoons chopped well-washed parsley

½ cup wheat germ

8 slices whole grain bread

Tofu, also called bean curd, is a great source of protein, and is lactose-free. It will remain fresh in the refrigerator for up to 1 week. See page 213 for rice-cooking instructions.

1. Preheat the oven to 350°F.

2. Place the tofu, rice, onion, eggs, salt, bread crumbs, paprika, and parsley in a large bowl, and mix thoroughly.

3. Place the wheat germ in a shallow bowl, or on a piece of wax paper. Form the tofu mixture into four patties, and roll in the wheat germ.

4. Coat a cookie sheet with nonstick cooking spray. Place the patties on the sheet, and bake for 35 minutes, or until heated through. Serve on the bread, and garnish as desired with lettuce, tomato, onion, or mustard.

NUTRITION INFORMATION (PER SERVING):
Calories: 550   Fat: 17 g   Carbohydrate: 73 g   Protein: 33 g

---

Good for constipation and weight gain.

Modification

If experiencing diarrhea or nausea and vomiting, omit the brown rice and wheat germ, and use 1 ½ cups white rice. Omit the onion, and use 1 teaspoon onion powder. Omit the eggs, and use 4 egg whites. Use white bread instead of whole wheat.

MODIFIED NUTRITION INFORMATION:
Calories: 480   Fat: 10 g   Carbohydrate: 75 g   Protein: 25 g

---

Tempting Treats

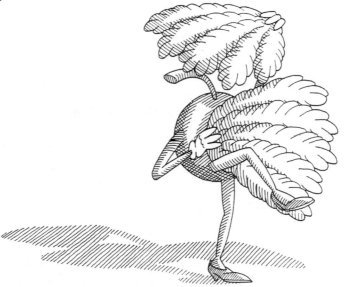

We've talked a great deal about limiting the amount of simple sugars and fat in your diet. This does not, however, mean that you must or should completely forego sweets. As long as you make sure to satisfy your overall nutrition requirements for the day, you should go ahead and indulge in the treat of your choice.

There are several ways to make dessert a healthy part of your diet. One is to use low-fat ingredients, such as yogurt and fruit, to add sweetness. Another is to use a variety of spices and flavorings, such as lemon peel, vanilla extract, and cinnamon, to perk up the flavor. And another is to use vegetables, notably carrots and zucchini, that are as at home on the dessert plate as they are on the dinner plate.

In this section, you will find a variety of tempting recipes. There are tasty cakes, such as Easy Carrot Cake and Lemon Gingerbread Cake. There are rich puddings, such as Colonial Apple Custard and Microwave Fruit Pudding. And there are other goodies, such as Chocolate Dreams (a taste-tester favorite) and No-Bake Cookies. You're sure to find something that will please your sweet tooth!

Recipe-by-Symptoms Chart

Different recipes in this section are designed to address different symptoms that commonly occur in people with HIV disease. This chart can help you find recipes to ease your symptoms. You'll note that some recipes address multiple symptoms.

ALTERATIONS IN TASTE	Apricot Fruit Bars, Blueberry Crisp, Colonial Apple Custard, Easy Apple Cake, Grandma Jarvie's Finnish Klapapuuroa, Lemon Cake, Lemon Gingerbread Cake, Microwave Fruit Pudding
CHEWING AND SWALLOWING DIFFICULTIES	Baked Rice Pudding, Banana Sweet Potato Pudding, Blueberry Crisp, Colonial Apple Custard, Custard Bread Pudding, Easy Carrot Cake, Grandma Jarvie's Finnish Klapapuuroa, Lemon Gingerbread Cake, Microwave Fruit Pudding, No-Bake Cookies, Zucchini Chocolate Cake
CONSTIPATION	Apricot Fruit Bars, Custard Bread Pudding, Microwave Fruit Pudding
DIARRHEA	Baked Rice Pudding (modified), Blueberry Crisp (modified), Custard Bread Pudding (modified), Easy Apple Cake (modified), Easy Carrot Cake, Grandma Jarvie's Finnish Klapapuuroa, Lemon Cake (modified), Tofu Cheesecake
DRY MOUTH	Baked Rice Pudding, Banana Sweet Potato Pudding, Colonial Apple Custard, Custard Bread Pudding, Grandma Jarvie's Finnish Klapapuuroa, Microwave Fruit Pudding
FATIGUE	Baked Rice Pudding, Banana Sweet Potato Pudding, Blueberry Crisp, Chocolate Dreams, Colonial Apple Custard, Custard Bread Pudding, Easy Apple Cake, Easy Carrot Cake, Graham and Peanut Butter Cookies, Microwave Fruit Pudding
LOSS OF APPETITE	Apricot Fruit Bars, Baked Rice Pudding, Banana Sweet Potato Pudding, Blueberry Crisp, Chocolate Dreams, Colonial Apple Custard, Easy Apple Cake, Easy Carrot Cake, Graham and Peanut Butter Cookies, Grandma Jarvie's Finnish Klapapuuroa, Lemon Cake, Lemon Gingerbread Cake, Microwave Fruit Pudding, No-Bake Cookies, Tofu Cheesecake

MOUTH AND THROAT SORES	Baked Rice Pudding (modified), Banana Sweet Potato Pudding, Chocolate Dreams, Colonial Apple Custard, Custard Bread Pudding, Easy Carrot Cake, Grandma Jarvie's Finnish Klapapuuroa, No-Bake Cookies, Tofu Cheesecake, Zucchini Chocolate Cake
NAUSEA AND VOMITING	Apricot Fruit Bars, Baked Rice Pudding (modified), Banana Sweet Potato Pudding, Blueberry Crisp, Custard Bread Pudding, Easy Apple Cake (modified), Easy Carrot Cake, Grandma Jarvie's Finnish Klapapuuroa, Lemon Cake (modified), Lemon Gingerbread Cake, Microwave Fruit Pudding
WEIGHT GAIN	Apricot Fruit Bars, Baked Rice Pudding, Chocolate Dreams, Colonial Apple Custard, Easy Apple Cake, Graham and Peanut Butter Cookies, Lemon Cake, No-Bake Cookies, Tofu Cheesecake, Zucchini Chocolate Cake

Easy Apple Cake

Yield: 8 servings
Preparation time: 20 minutes
to assemble; 45 to 50 minutes
to bake

1 egg, beaten

2 cups cubed well-washed apple

1 cup sugar

¼ cup canola oil

1 teaspoon vanilla extract

½ cup chopped walnuts

½ cup raisins

1 cup white flour

1 teaspoon baking soda

2 teaspoons ground cinnamon

Try this cake dusted with powdered sugar, or topped with ice cream or vanilla low-fat yogurt.

1. Preheat the oven to 350°F.

2. Place the egg and apple in a large bowl, and mix thoroughly. Add the sugar, oil, vanilla, walnuts, and raisins, and mix again.

3. Place the remaining ingredients in a separate bowl, and mix thoroughly. Add to the apple mixture, and mix again.

4. Coat an 8-inch square baking dish with nonstick cooking spray, and flour the dish. Pour the batter into the dish, and bake for 45 to 50 minutes, or until the cake is firm to the touch and an inserted knife or toothpick comes out clean. Cool the cake in the pan. Serve either warm or cool.

NUTRITION INFORMATION (PER SERVING):
Calories: 310   Fat: 12 g   Carbohydrate: 50 g   Protein: 4 g

---

Good for alterations in taste, fatigue,
loss of appetite, and weight gain.

Modification

If experiencing diarrhea or nausea and vomiting, peel the apples, and use 3 cups of apples instead of 2. Omit the egg, and use 2 egg whites. Omit the oil, and use $\frac{1}{4}$ cup applesauce. Omit nuts and raisins.

MODIFIED NUTRITION INFORMATION:
Calories: 190   Fat: 1 g   Carbohydrate: 46 g   Protein: 3 g

Easy Carrot Cake

Yield: 8 servings
Preparation time: 15 minutes
to assemble; 25 to 30 minutes
to bake

1 cup white flour

1 cup sugar

½ teaspoon baking soda

1 teaspoon ground cinnamon

½ cup applesauce

4 egg whites, beaten

2 cups grated carrot, lightly
   packed (about 4
   medium-sized carrots)

This carrot cake is both easy to make and easy to digest.

1. Preheat the oven to 350°F.

2. Place all the ingredients in a large bowl, and mix thoroughly.

3. Coat a 9-inch square baking dish with nonstick cooking spray, and flour the dish. Pour the batter into the baking dish, and bake for 25 to 30 minutes, or until the cake is firm to the touch and an inserted knife or toothpick comes out clean. Cool the cake in the pan. Serve plain, or sprinkle some powdered sugar over the top.

NUTRITION INFORMATION (PER SERVING):

Calories: 175   Fat: 1 g   Carbohydrate: 41 g   Protein: 4 g

Good for chewing and swallowing difficulties, diarrhea, fatigue, loss of appetite, mouth and throat sores, and nausea and vomiting.

Tofu Cheesecake

Yield: 8 servings
Preparation time: 10 minutes to
assemble; 40 minutes to bake

1 ½ pounds light soft tofu,
   drained

½ cup sugar

1 tablespoon vanilla extract

2 tablespoons lemon juice

1 teaspoon ground cinnamon

1 tablespoon freshly grated
   lemon peel

1 9-inch graham cracker crust

Tofu makes this lactose-free cake more nutritious than traditional cheese-cake.

1. Preheat the oven to 350°F.

2. Place all ingredients except the crust in a blender, and blend until smooth.

3. Pour the mixture into the pie crust, and bake for about 40 minutes, or until the cake is firm to the touch. Cool it in the refrigerator. Top with fruit, if desired.

NUTRITION INFORMATION (PER SERVING):

Calories: 240   Fat: 8 g   Carbohydrate: 30 g   Protein: 13 g

---

Good for diarrhea, loss of appetite, mouth and throat sores, and weight gain.

Lemon Cake

Yield: 8 servings
Preparation time: 15 minutes
to assemble; 40 to 45 minutes
to bake

½ cup butter

⅔ cup sugar

2 eggs

1 cup white flour

¼ teaspoon baking powder

1 tablespoon freshly grated
lemon peel

1 tablespoon lemon juice

ICING

¼ cup butter

2 teaspoons lemon juice,
preferably fresh-squeezed

⅔ cup powdered sugar

The tart taste of lemon gives this cake a special zing.

1. Preheat the oven to 350°F.

2. Place all the batter ingredients in a large bowl, and beat until well blended.

3. Coat an 8-inch round cake pan with nonstick cooking spray, and flour the pan. Pour the batter into the pan. Bake for 40 to 45 minutes, or until the cake is firm to the touch and an inserted knife or toothpick comes out clean. Cool the cake in the pan.

4. To make the icing, place all the icing ingredients in a small bowl, and beat together. Spread over the top of the cooled cake.

NUTRITION INFORMATION (PER SERVING):

Calories: 320   Fat: 19 g   Carbohydrate: 37 g   Protein: 3 g

---

Good for alterations in taste, loss of appetite, and weight gain.

Modification

If experiencing diarrhea or nausea and vomiting, omit the eggs, and use four egg whites. Omit the butter, and use ½ cup applesauce. For the icing, omit the butter, and use 2 tablespoons margarine, and increase the lemon juice used from 2 teaspoons to 1 tablespoon.

MODIFIED NUTRITION INFORMATION:

Calories: 190   Fat: 3 g   Carbohydrate: 38 g   Protein: 3 g

Lemon Gingerbread Cake

Yield: 9 servings
Preparation time: 20 minutes to
assemble; 25 minutes to bake

2 tablespoons sugar

2 tablespoons butter

2 teaspoons freshly grated
  lemon peel

1 egg white

1 cup white flour

½ cup whole wheat flour

½ teaspoon baking soda

¼ teaspoon salt

½ teaspoon ground ginger

1 teaspoon ground cinnamon

½ cup low-fat buttermilk (see
  page 103)

½ cup dark molasses

2 teaspoons powdered sugar

Lemon and ginger combine to make this cake a good stomach-soother.

1. Preheat the oven to 350°F.

2. Place the sugar and butter in a large bowl, and cream until fluffy. Add the lemon peel and egg white, and beat until blended.

3. Place the flours, baking soda, salt, ginger, and cinnamon in a separate bowl, and mix thoroughly.

4. Place the buttermilk and molasses in a third bowl, and blend.

5. Gradually add the flour mixture and then the buttermilk mixture to the sugar mixture, stirring between each addition.

6. Coat an 8-inch square baking dish with nonstick cooking spray, and flour the dish. Pour the batter into the dish, and bake for 25 minutes, or until the cake is firm to the touch and an inserted knife or toothpick comes out clean. Cool completely on a wire rack before removing from the pan. Sprinkle with the powdered sugar.

NUTRITION INFORMATION (PER SERVING):
Calories: 160　　Fat: 3 g　　Carbohydrate: 30 g　　Protein: 3 g

Good for alterations in taste, chewing and swallowing difficulties,
loss of appetite, and nausea and vomiting.

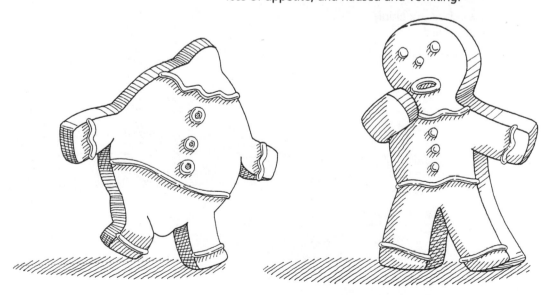

Zucchini Chocolate Cake

Yield: 12 servings
Preparation time: 20 minutes
to assemble; 35 to 40 minutes
to bake

¼ cup butter, softened

¼ cup canola oil

¼ cup plain low-fat yogurt

1 ¾ cups sugar

½ cup sour milk (1 teaspoon lemon juice plus ½ cup low-fat milk)

1 egg plus 2 egg whites

1 teaspoon vanilla extract

2 ½ cups white flour

⅓ cup unsweetened cocoa powder

½ teaspoon baking powder

1 teaspoon baking soda

½ teaspoon ground cinnamon

½ teaspoon ground cloves

2 cups well-washed zucchini, peeled and grated

¼ cup chocolate chips

Vegetables such as zucchini are tasty additions to cakes. This delicious cake proves it!

1. Preheat the oven to 325°F.

2. Place the butter, oil, yogurt, and sugar in a large bowl, and cream together. Add the milk, eggs, and vanilla, and blend.

3. Place the flour, cocoa, baking powder, baking soda, cinnamon, and cloves in a separate bowl, and mix thoroughly.

4. Add the butter mixture to the flour mixture, and mix thoroughly. Add the zucchini, and mix again.

5. Coat a 9-x-13-inch baking dish with nonstick cooking spray, and flour the dish. Pour the batter into the baking dish, and top with the chocolate chips. Bake for 35 to 40 minutes, or until the cake is firm to the touch and an inserted knife or toothpick comes out clean. Cool the cake in the pan.

NUTRITION INFORMATION (PER SERVING):

Calories: 320   Fat: 10 g   Carbohydrate: 54 g   Protein: 5 g

---

Good for chewing and swallowing difficulties,
mouth and throat sores, and weight gain.

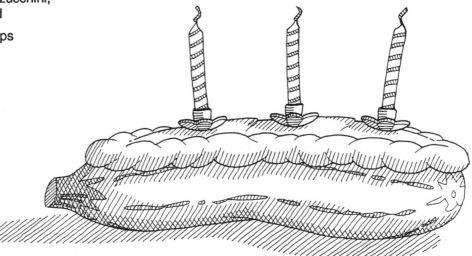

Banana Sweet Potato Pudding

Yield: 4 servings
Preparation time: 15 minutes to assemble; 45 minutes to bake

2 ripe bananas, mashed

1 cup plain low-fat yogurt

½ teaspoon salt

¼ cup raisins

1 cup mashed, cooked sweet potato

2 tablespoons brown sugar

2 egg yolks, slightly beaten

Sweet potatoes for dessert? You bet! If you're not sure how to cook the sweet potatoes, see page 178.

1. Preheat the oven to 300°F.

2. Place all of the ingredients in a large bowl, and mix thoroughly.

3. Coat an 8-inch square baking dish with nonstick cooking spray. Spoon the mixture into the dish, and bake for 45 minutes, or until the pudding is set and browned on top. Serve warm or chilled.

NUTRITION INFORMATION (PER SERVING):

Calories: 260   Fat: 4 g   Carbohydrate: 51 g   Protein: 7 g

Good for chewing and swallowing difficulties, dry mouth, fatigue, loss of appetite, mouth and throat sores, and nausea and vomiting.

Colonial Apple Custard

Yield: 2 servings
Preparation time: 15 minutes to assemble; 30 minutes to bake

1 tablespoon melted butter

1 cup applesauce

3 eggs, beaten

½ teaspoon salt

1 teaspoon vanilla extract

½ teaspoon ground nutmeg

This traditional custard makes both a great dessert and a wonderful snack.

1. Preheat the oven to 350°F.

2. Place the butter, applesauce, eggs, salt, and vanilla in a medium-sized bowl, and blend.

3. Coat four custard cups with nonstick cooking spray. Pour the custard into the cups, and sprinkle with the nutmeg. Place the cups in a pan with 2 inches of water in the bottom, and bake for 30 minutes—an inserted knife or toothpick should come out clean. Serve warm or chilled.

NUTRITION INFORMATION (PER SERVING):

Calories: 230   Fat: 14 g   Carbohydrate: 16 g   Protein: 10 g

---

Good for alterations in taste, chewing and swallowing difficulties, dry mouth, fatigue, loss of appetite, mouth and throat sores, and weight gain.

Custard Bread Pudding

Yield: 6 servings
Preparation time: 15 minutes
to assemble; 30 to 35 minutes
to bake

8 slices whole wheat bread

2 ⅔ cups evaporated skim milk

6 egg whites

⅓ cup honey

1 teaspoon vanilla extract

1 teaspoon ground cinnamon

½ teaspoon ground nutmeg

This is a delicious way to use bread that's gone a little stale.

1. Preheat the oven to 375°F.

2. Coat a 9-inch square baking dish with nonstick cooking spray. Line the bottom of the dish with 4 bread slices.

3. Place the milk, egg whites, honey, vanilla, and cinnamon in a large bowl, and beat together using a wire whisk.

4. Pour half of the milk mixture over the bread slices in the dish. Cover with the 4 remaining bread slices, and pour in the remaining custard. Sprinkle with the nutmeg.

5. Bake for 30 to 35 minutes, or until the custard is set. Serve warm or chilled.

NUTRITION INFORMATION (PER SERVING):

Calories: 265   Fat: 3 g   Carbohydrate: 44 g   Protein: 14 g

---

Good for chewing and swallowing difficulties, constipation, dry mouth, fatigue, mouth and throat sores, and nausea and vomiting.

Modification

If experiencing diarrhea, omit the whole wheat bread, and use white bread. Omit the evaporated milk, and use 2 ⅔ cups light soymilk or lactose-reduced milk.

MODIFIED NUTRITION INFORMATION:

Calories: 195   Fat: 3 g   Carbohydrate: 33 g   Protein: 9 g

Grandma Jarvie's
Finnish Klapapuuroa

Yield: 4 servings
Preparation time: 20 minutes

3 cups grape juice

⅓ cup dry wheat farina

This Old World dessert has the consistency of pudding.

1. Place the juice in a medium-sized saucepan over high heat, and bring to a boil.

2. Stir in the farina, reduce the heat to low, and continue to cook, stirring constantly, for 10 minutes.

3. Pour the hot pudding into a small bowl, beat until light and fluffy, about 10 minutes. Serve hot, topped with low-fat yogurt and whipped topping.

NUTRITION INFORMATION (PER SERVING):

Calories: 140   Fat: 1 g   Carbohydrate: 33 g   Protein: 2 g

Good for alterations in taste, chewing and swallowing difficulties, diarrhea, dry mouth, loss of appetite, mouth and throat sores, and nausea and vomiting.

Chocolate Dreams

Yield: 24 dreams
Preparation time: 20 minutes to assemble; 1 hour to freeze

1 package (4 ounces) chocolate-flavored instant pudding

2 cups low-fat milk, chilled

½ cup creamy peanut butter

48 graham crackers, 4½-x- 2 ½-inch

Caution: Make this recipe once, and you'll be hooked! Our tasters refused to try anything else until we promised to make more of these addictive treats.

1. Place the pudding, milk, and peanut butter in a large bowl, and mix thoroughly.

2. Spread a heaping teaspoonful of the mixture on a graham cracker, and top with another cracker. Repeat until all of the pudding mixture has been used.

3. Place the dreams in a sealed container, and freeze at least 1 hour.

NUTRITION INFORMATION (PER DREAM):

Calories: 115   Fat: 4 g   Carbohydrate: 16 g   Protein: 3 g

Good for fatigue, loss of appetite, mouth and throat sores, and weight gain.

Microwave Fruit Pudding

Yield: 6 servings
Preparation time: 35 minutes to assemble; 1 hour to chill

1 package (6 ounces) vanilla pudding

4 cups low-fat milk

1 can (15 ounces) pineapple chunks in juice, drained (reserve juice)

1 can (5 ounces) mandarin oranges, drained (reserve juice)

2 ripe bananas, sliced

½ cup pitted and halved well-washed cherries

This is a refreshing summertime treat.

1. Prepare the pudding according to the package directions, using the milk. Pour the pudding into a microwave-safe 1 ½-quart dish.

2. Pour the pineapple juice into a measuring cup, and add enough mandarin orange juice to make 1 cup. Stir the combined juices into the pudding.

3. Microwave the pudding mixture on high power for 3 to 4 minutes, or until mixture boils, stirring twice.

4. Add the pineapple chunks and oranges, and refrigerate for 1 hour. Just before serving, mix in the bananas and garnish with the cherries.

NUTRITION INFORMATION (PER SERVING):
Calories: 285   Fat: 4 g   Carbohydrate: 60 g   Protein: 7 g

Good for alterations in taste, chewing and swallowing difficulties, constipation, dry mouth, fatigue, loss of appetite, and nausea and vomiting.

Baked Rice Pudding

Yield: 4 servings
Preparation time: 15 minutes to assemble; 30 minutes to bake

2 cups cooked brown rice

½ cup raisins

½ teaspoon freshly grated lemon peel

1 teaspoon lemon juice

½ cup honey

½ teaspoon vanilla extract

3 eggs

2 ½ cups low-fat milk

¼ teaspoon salt

You may find that this batter is watery prior to baking, but it firms up nicely. See page 213 for rice-cooking instructions.

1. Preheat the oven to 350°F.

2. Place the rice, raisins, lemon peel, and juice in a medium-sized bowl, and mix thoroughly.

3. Coat an 8-inch square baking dish with nonstick cooking spray. Pour the rice mixture into the dish.

4. Place the remaining ingredients in a large bowl, and beat together. Pour over the rice mixture. Bake for 30 minutes, or until the pudding is set. Serve warm or chilled.

NUTRITION INFORMATION (PER SERVING):

Calories: 425   Fat: 8 g   Carbohydrate: 80 g   Protein: 13 g

Good for chewing and swallowing difficulties, dry mouth,
fatigue, loss of appetite, and weight gain.

Modifications

If experiencing diarrhea or nausea and vomiting, omit the brown
rice, and use white rice. Omit the raisins. Omit the low-fat milk, and
use 2 $\frac{1}{2}$ cups soymilk or lactose-reduced milk. Omit the 3 eggs,
and use 1 whole egg and 4 egg whites.

MODIFIED NUTRITION INFORMATION:

Calories: 350   Fat: 4 g   Carbohydrate: 67 g   Protein: 12 g

If experiencing mouth and throat sores, omit the lemon juice and
peel. The nutrition information doesn't change.

Graham and Peanut Butter Cookies

Yield: 12 cookies
Preparation time: 25 minutes to
assemble; 10 minutes to bake

1 ¼ cups graham cracker
crumbs

1 teaspoon baking powder

1 egg, lightly beaten

3 tablespoon water

2 tablespoons creamy peanut
butter

½ teaspoon vanilla extract

There is no sugar or flour in this recipe.

1. Preheat the oven to 350°F.

2. Place the cracker crumbs and baking powder in a medium-sized bowl,
and mix thoroughly. Add the remaining ingredients, and mix until well
blended. Let the mixture stand for 5 minutes, then roll the dough into 12
balls.

3. Coat a cookie sheet with nonstick cooking spray. Place the balls on
the cookie sheet, and flatten slightly with a fork dipped in cold water.

4. Bake for approximately 10 minutes, or until lightly browned. Let stand
for 5 minutes, then transfer to a wire rack for cooling.

NUTRITION INFORMATION (PER COOKIE):

Calories: 78   Fat: 3 g   Carbohydrate: 10 g   Protein: 2 g

Good for fatigue, loss of appetite, and weight gain.

Apricot Fruit Bars

Yield: 9 bars
*Preparation time: 25 minutes
to assemble; 30 to 35 minutes
to bake*

½ cup plain low-fat yogurt

⅔ cup sugar

¼ cup evaporated skim milk

1 cup plus 2 tablespoons whole
   wheat flour, divided

½ teaspoon baking powder

1 cup rolled oats

¼ cup wheat germ

¾ cup chopped dried fruit

½ cup apricot preserves

If you crave something chewy and sweet, make up a batch of these fruit bars.

1. Preheat the oven to 350°F.

2. Place the yogurt, sugar, and milk in a large bowl, and blend. Place 1 cup of the flour in a separate bowl, add the baking powder, oats, and wheat germ, and mix thoroughly. Add the yogurt mixture to the dry ingredients, and mix again.

3. Place the dried fruit in a separate bowl, and sprinkle with the remaining 2 tablespoons of flour. Add the apricot preserves, and mix thoroughly.

4. Coat an 8-inch square baking dish with nonstick cooking spray. Spread half of the yogurt mixture in the bottom of the baking dish. Spoon in the fruit mixture, and top with the rest of the yogurt mixture. Bake for 30 to 35 minutes, or until firm. Cool completely in the pan before cutting into bars.

NUTRITION INFORMATION (PER BAR):
Calories: 250   Fat: 2 g   Carbohydrate: 56 g   Protein: 6 g

Good for alterations in taste, constipation, loss of appetite,
nausea and vomiting, and weight gain.

Blueberry Crisp

Yield: 6 servings
Preparation time: 10 minutes to assemble; 30 minutes to bake

3 cups blueberries,
   well-washed fresh or thawed
   frozen

2 tablespoons lemon juice

⅔ cup brown sugar, firmly
   packed

1 tablespoon white flour

½ cup quick-cooking oats

1 teaspoon ground cinnamon

½ teaspoon salt

2 tablespoons butter

This is the perfect end to a good meal.

1. Preheat the oven to 375°F.

2. Coat an 8-inch square baking dish with nonstick cooking spray. Spread the blueberries in the bottom of the baking dish, and sprinkle with the lemon juice.

3. Place the sugar, flour, oats, cinnamon, and salt in a small bowl, and mix thoroughly. Spread over the blueberries. Dot the top evenly with the butter. Bake for 30 minutes, or until heated through and the crust is lightly browned. Cool in the pan.

NUTRITION INFORMATION (PER SERVING):

Calories: 200   Fat: 5 g   Carbohydrate: 40 g   Protein: 2 g

Good for alterations in taste, chewing and swallowing difficulties, fatigue, loss of appetite, and nausea and vomiting.

Modification

If experiencing diarrhea, omit the butter and use margarine. The nutrition information doesn't change.

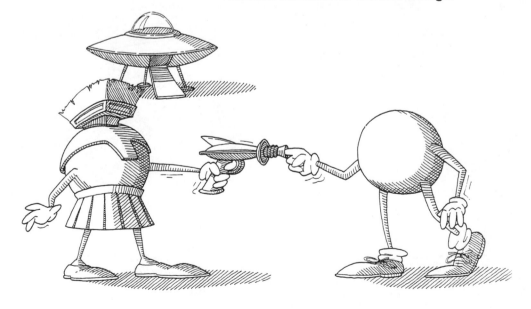

No-Bake Cookies

Yield: 36 cookies
Preparation time: 15 minutes to prepare; 1 hour to chill

2 cups sugar

¼ cup nonfat dry milk powder

½ cup water

½ cup butter

⅓ cup unsweetened cocoa powder

3 cups rolled oats

½ cup creamy peanut butter

1 teaspoon vanilla extract

Who needs an oven to make cookies? These treats harden as they cool.

1. Place the sugar, milk powder, water, and butter in a medium-sized saucepan over medium heat, and cook until the sugar is dissolved and the mixture begins to bubble.

2. Place the remaining ingredients in a large bowl, and mix thoroughly. Pour the sugar mixture into the bowl, and blend.

3. Drop the mixture by the tablespoonful onto a sheet of wax paper. Cool in the refrigerator for 1 hour. When hardened, place in an airtight container and store for up to 2 weeks in the refrigerator. Or, freeze for up to 3 months.

NUTRITION INFORMATION (PER COOKIE):
Calories: 115   Fat: 5 g   Carbohydrate: 17 g   Protein: 2 g

Good for chewing and swallowing difficulties, loss of appetite, mouth and throat sores, and weight gain.

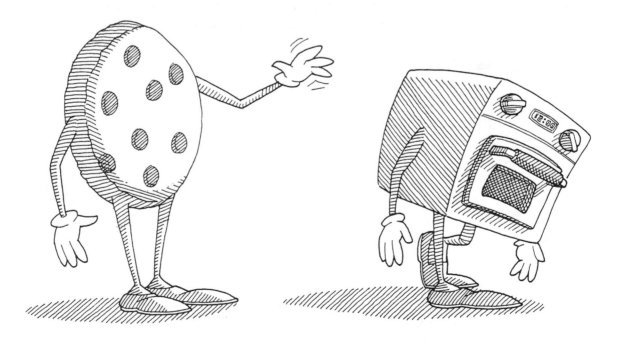

Resource List

BOOKS AND PERIODICALS

Food Sensitivity Series
American Dietetic Association
216 West Jackson
Suite 800
Chicago IL 60606-6955
1-800-366-1655

*Covers food sensitivity, gluten intolerance,
and lactose intolerance.*

The Honest Herbal—A Sensible Guide
to the Use of Herbs and Related Remedies
Varro E. Tyler, Ph.D.
Pharmaceutical Products Press
10 Alice Street
Binghamton NY 13904-1580

Nutrition Action Health Newsletter
Center for Science in the Public Interest
1875 Connecticut Avenue NW
Suite 300
Washington DC 20009
202-332-9110

Positive Nutrition: A Nutrition and HIV Newsletter
Project Open Hand
2720 17th Street
San Francisco CA 94110
415-558-0600

University of California at Berkeley
Wellness Encyclopedia of Food and Nutrition
S. Margen and the Editors of the University
of California at Berkeley Wellness Letter
Published by Rebus, 1992 (New York).
Distributed by Random House.

University of California at Berkeley Wellness Letter
Subscription Department
P.O. Box 420148
Palm Coast FL 32142
904-445-6414

The Wellness Guide to Lifelong Fitness
T. White and the Editors of the University
of California at Berkeley Wellness Letter
Published by Rebus, 1993 (New York).
Distributed by Random House.

REFERRALS

American Dietetic Association
Center for Nutrition and Dietetics
Consumer Nutrition Hotline
1-800-366-1655

*This service can answsr your food and nutrition
questions, and can refer you to a registered dietitian
in your area.*

CDC National AIDS Clearinghouse
Document Delivery Service
P.O. Box 6003
Rockville MD 20849-6003
1-800-458-5231

*This service can provide you with a detailed list
of most of the published material on HIV
and nutrition, and with a list of HIV agencies
and services throughout the country.*

CDC National AIDS Hotline
- 1-800-342-AIDS
- 1-800-344-SIDA (Spanish)
- 1-800-AIDS-TTY (for the hearing-impaired)
- 713-524-2437—Houston
- 202-332-AIDS—Washington DC

*Also contact your local health department for
referrals to registered dietitians, nutrition
and meal programs, and other HIV services
in your community.*

References

Abrams B, Duncan D, and Hertz-Picciotto I. A Prospective Study of Dietary Intake and Acquired Immune Deficiency Syndrome in HIV-Seropositive Homosexual Men. *Journal of Acquired Immune Deficiency Syndromes* 6:949–958, 1993.

Anastasi J and Sun Lee V. HIV Wasting: How to Stop the Cycle. *American Journal of Nutrition*, June 1994, 18–25.

Coodley GO. Update on Vitamins, Minerals, and the Carotenoids. *Journal of the Physicians Association for AIDS Care*, January 1995, 24–29.

Coodley GO, Loveless MO, and Merrill TM. The HIV Wasting Syndrome: A Review. *Journal of Acquired Immune Deficiency Syndromes* 7:681–694, 1994.

Cope FO. The Role of Nutrition in AIDS Management. *Journal of the International Association of Physicians in AIDS Care*, July 1995, 26–29.

Fields-Gardner C. Food-Based Nutrients as Therapeutic Options In HIV Care. *Bulletin of Experimental Treatments for AIDS*, September 1994, 44–46.

Fields-Gardner C. Vitamin and Mineral Megadosing as an Alternative Therapy. *Community Prescription Service Info Pack* 4(1):4–6, Spring 1995.

Galvin TA. Micronutrients: Implications in Human Immunodeficiency Virus Disease. *Topics in Clinical Nutrition* 7(3):63–73, 1992.

Gilden D. Nutritional Intervention in HIV Disease. *Bulletin of Experimental Treatments for AIDS*, March 1994, 3–11.

Guenter P, Nuurahainen N, Simons G, Kosok A, Cohan G, Rudenstein R, and Turner J. Relationships Among Nutritional Status, Disease Progression, and Survival in HIV Infection. *Journal of Acquired Immune Deficiency Syndromes* 6:1130–1138, 1993.

Hellerstein MK, Kahn J, Mudie H, and Viteri F. Current Approach to the Treatment of Human Immunodeficiency Virus-Associated Weight Loss: Pathophysiologic Considerations and Emerging Management Strategies. *Seminars in Oncology* 17(6, Suppl 9):17–33, December 1990.

Jarvie J. and Brauer J. Vitamins, Minerals and HIV Disease. *Positive Nutrition* 4:1,6, Winter 1994.

Keusch GT and Thea D. Malnutrition in AIDS. *Clinical Nutrition* 77(4):795–809, July 1993.

Kotler DP. Pathophysiology of Malnutrition. *Journal*

of the Physicians Association for AIDS Care, October 1993, 402–405.

Kotler DP. Malnutrition. *Critical Path AIDS Project* 29:1–13, Summer 1994.

Kotler DP. HIV-Associated Malnutrition. *Journal of the Physicians Association for AIDS Care*, January 1995, 12–15.

Kotler DP, Tierney A, Branner S, Couteure S, Wang J, and Pierson R. Preservation of Short-term Energy Balance in Clinically Stable Patients with AIDS. *American Journal of Clinical Nutrition* 51:7–13, 1990.

Lein B. Nutrition and Wasting. *Bulletin of Experimental Treatments for AIDS*, December 1994, 37–40.

Margen S and the Editors of the University of California at Berkeley Wellness Letter. *University of California at Berkeley Wellness Encyclopedia of Food and Nutrition.* New York: Rebus, 1992. Distributed by Random House.

McKinley M, Goodman-Block J, Lesser M, and Salbe A. Improved Body Weight Status as a Result of Nutrition Intervention in Adult, HIV-Positive Outpatients. *Journal of the American Dietetic Association* 94(9):1014–1017, September 1994.

McMillan L. The Dairy Dilemma. *Positive Nutrition* 3:6, 8, Fall 1993.

Timbo BB and Tollefson L. Nutrition: A Cofactor in HIV Disease. *Journal of American Dietetic Association* 94:1019–1022, September 1994.

Udine L and Capozza C. Nutritional Care of the HIV Client. *Caring Magazine*, May 1993, 36–40.

United States Department of Health and Human Services, Public Health Service, National Institutes of Health. *Understanding the Immune System.* NIH Publication No. 90–529, March 1990.

Watson R. Supplemental Vitamin A and E: Will AIDS Patients Benefit? *Nutrition and the M.D.* 21(3):1–3, March 1995.

White T and the Editors of the University of California at Berkeley Wellness Letter. *The Wellness Guide to Lifelong Fitness.* New York: Rebus 1993. Distributed by Random House.

Index